AF334180

GI Endoscopy – Standards and Innovations

FALK SYMPOSIUM 166

GI Endoscopy – Standards and Innovations

Edited by

C Ell
Dr Horst Schmidt Clinic
Wiesbaden
Germany

T Ponchon
Eduard Herriot Hospital
Lyon
France

JF Riemann
Clinical Centre
Ludwigsghafen
Germany

P Sakai
University of São Paulo
São Paulo
Brazil

H Yamamoto
Jichi Medical School
Tochigi
Japan

Proceedings of the Falk Symposium 166 held in
Mainz, Germany
September 18–19, 2008

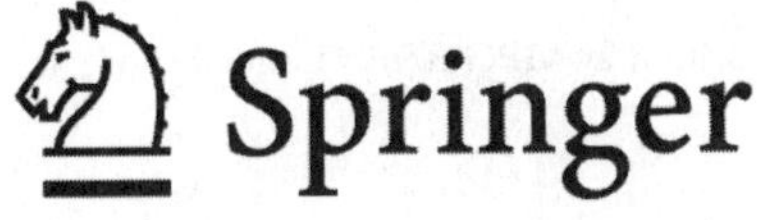

Library of Congress Cataloging-in-Publication Data is available.

ISBN 978-90-481-2748-1

Published by Springer,
PO Box 17, 3300 AA Dordrecht, The Netherlands

Sold and distributed in North, Central and South America
by Springer,
101 Philip Drive, Norwell, MA 02061 USA

In all other countries, sold and distributed
by Springer,
PO Box 322, 3300 AH Dordrecht, The Netherlands

Printed on acid-free paper

Contents

CONTENTS

List of principal contributors

B Dallemagne
Hôpitaux Universitaires
IRCA/EITS Institute
1, Place de l'Hopital
67091 Strasbourg
France

CF Dietrich
Department of Gastroenterology
Innere Medizin II
Caritas Krankenhaus
Uhlandstr. 7
97980 Bad Mergentheim
Germany

D Hartmann
Medizinische Klinik C
Klinikum der Stadt Ludwigshafen
  GmbH
Bremserstr. 79
67063 Ludwigshafen
Germany

A May
Innere Medizin II
HSK, Dr Horst Schmidt Klinik
Ludwig-Erhard-Str. 100
65199 Wiesbaden
Germany

J Pohl
Innere Medizin II
HSK Dr Horst Schmidt Klinik
Ludwig-Erhard Str. 100
65199 Wiesbaden
Germany

T Ponchon
Hôpital Eduard Herriot
Specialités Digestives
Pavillon H
Place d'Arsonval
69437 Lyon
France

J Regula
Maria Sklodowska-Curie Memorial
  Cancer Centre
Medical Centre for Postgraduate
  Education
Department of Gastroenterology
Roentgen Street 5
02-781 Warsaw
Poland

JF Riemann
c/o Stiftung LebensBlicke
Klinikum der Stadt Ludwigshafen
Bremserstr. 79
67063 Ludwigshafen
Germany

P Sakai
Hospital das Clinicas
Universidade de São Paulo
Gastrointestinal Unit
Rua Joao Juliao 331
01323-02 São Paulo
Brazil

B Schumacher
EVK Evangelisches Krankenhaus
Kirchfeldstr. 40
40217 Düsseldorf
Germany

G Triadafilopoulos
Stanford University School of
  Medicine
Department of Gastroenterology and
  Hepatology
300 Pasteur Drive
Stanford, CA 94305
USA

P Vilmann
Department of Surgical
  Gastroenterology
Gentofte University Hospital
Niels Andersens vej 65
2900 Hellerup
Denmark

H Yamamoto
Jichi Medical University
Department of Endoscopic Research
  and International Education
3311-1 Yakushiji, Shimotsuke
Tochigi 329-0498
Japan

List of chairpersons

D Coumaros
Nouvel Hôpital Civil
Hôpitaux Universitaires
Pole Hépato-Digestif
1, Place de l'Hôpital
67091 Strasbourg
France

Z Döbrönte
Markusovszky Hospital
II Department of Medicine
Markusovszky u. 3
9700 Szombathely
Hungary

C Ell
Innere Medizin II
HSK Dr. Horst Schmidt Klinik
Ludwig-Erhard-Str. 100
65199 Wiesbaden
Germany

G Gay
Hôpitaux de Brabois
C.H.U. de Nancy
Departement de Medicine Interne
A Orientation Digestive
Allee du Morvan
54511 Vandoeuvre-Nancy
France

L Gossner
Innere Medizin I
Städtisches Klinikum
Moltkestr. 90
76133 Karlsruhe
Germany

F Hagenmüller
Innere Medizin I
Asklepios Klinik Altona
Paul-Ehrlich-Str. 1
22763 Hamburg
Germany

M Jung
Innere Medizin
Katholisches Klinikum Mainz
St. Hildegardis-Krankenhaus
Hildegardstr. 2
55131 Mainz
Germany

R Kiesslich
Innere Medizin I
Klinikum der Universität
Langenbeckstr. 1
55131 Mainz
Germany

D Lorenz
Allgemein-Viszeralchirurgie
HSK Dr. Horst Schmidt Klinik
Ludwig-Erhard-Str. 100
65199 Wiesbaden
Germany

PN Meier
Gastroenterologie
Diakoniekrankenhaus
Henriettenstiftung
Schwemannstr. 17
30559 Hannover
Germany

C Meyenberger
Kantonsspital
FMH Gastroenterologie
Rorschacherstr. 95
9007 St. Gallen
Switzerland

CJJ Mulder
Free University
Medical Center
Department of Gastroenterology
PO Box 7057
1007 MB Amsterdam
The Netherlands

A Pap
Orszagos Onkologiai Intezet
II. Department of Medicine
Rath György u. 7-9
1122 Budapest
Hungary

T Rabenstein
Gastroenterologie
Diakonissen-Stiftungs-Krankenhaus
Haus Hilgardstrasse
Hilgardstr. 26
67346 Speyer
Germany

A Repici
Istituto Clinico Humanitas
Department of Digestive Endoscopy
Via Manzoni 56
20089 Rozzano
Italy

R Schöfl
Krankenhaus der Elisabethinen
Gastroenterologie/Hepatologie
Fadingerstrasse 1
4010 Linz
Austria

H-J Schulz
Innere Medizin
Sana-Klinikum Lichtenberg
Oskar-Ziethen-Krankenhaus
Fanningerstr. 32
10365 Berlin
Germany

PD Siersema
Academisch Ziekenhuis Utrecht
Afd. Gastroenterologie
Heidelberglaan 100
3584 CX Utrecht
The Netherlands

SJ Spechler
VA Medical Center
Department of Gastroenterology
4500 S. Lancaster Road
Dallas, TX 75216-7167
USA

T Toyonaga
Kishiwada Tokushukai Hospital
Department of Gastroenterology
4-27-1 Kamori-cho, Kashiwada
Osaka 596-8522
Japan

GNJ Tytgat
Emeritus
Diepenbrockstr. 52
1077 WB Amsterdam
The Netherlands

Preface

Gastrointestinal (GI) endoscopy has become one of the most important techniques in the diagnosis and treatment of GI diseases. Flexible endoscopy together with chip technology has replaced many other diagnostic procedures as well as non-surgical and surgical therapeutic modalities within the last 30 years. GI endoscopy has achieved tremendous usage worldwide with more than one million procedures per day. Therefore, it is time to define standards for all these techniques as an orientation for less experienced endoscopists and in order to have an optimal tool for quality assessment.

Although the history of GI endoscopy covers a couple of decades, even in the last few years there have been new inventions which have enhanced the importance of GI endoscopy. Especially the mid-GI tract has been explored by endoscopic techniques such as capsule endoscopy and double balloon enteroscopy. Both have become milestones in GI endoscopy as well as endoscopic intraluminal resection of early cancer.

The Falk Symposium 166 brought together many leading endoscopists from all over the world to present and to discuss standards and innovations in excellent lectures, as well as in a two-day live course from the HSK Wiesbaden.

It was a great pleasure for me and the other scientific chairs to organize this symposium and the syllabus, which summarizes all important contributions.

C. Ell, Wiesbaden
T. Ponchon, Lyon
J. F. Riemann, Ludwigshafen
P. Sakai, Sao Paulo
H. Yamamoto, Tochigi

Section I
Oesophagus

Chair: L GOSSNER and SJ SPECHLER

1
Oesophagus: standards

P. SAKAI

PART 1: ZENKER'S DIVERTICULUM

Pharyngo-oesophageal diverticulum, also known as Zenker's diverticulum (ZD), is an acquired disease formed by the outpouching of hypopharyngeal mucosa between the inferior pharyngeal constrictor muscle and the cricopharyngeal muscle in an area of junctional muscle weakness known as Killian's triangle. Its pathophysiology is not well known but is thought to be incoordination between pharyngeal contraction and upper oesophageal sphincter relaxation. Evidence also suggests that, during swallowing, high hypopharyngeal pressures occur in some individuals because of poor compliance with the upper oesophageal sphincter[1]. As a result of this increased pressure, pharyngeal mucosa and submucosa bulge through this weakened area. In the early stages, outpouching of the mucosa may be reversible and may actually recede during muscle relaxation. In the later stages the diverticulum progressively enlarges and descends into the neck, most commonly on the left side. In some cases it may even extend down into the superior mediastinum.

Surgical treatment of ZD is a well-established modality and effective in 80–100% of patients. The preferred approach involves the resection of the pouch (diverticulectomy) plus cricopharyngeal myotomy through a left cervicotomy[2]. However, morbidity and mortality rates of this surgery are significant, mainly due to the advanced age of the patients involved and several comorbidities. Despite these factors, in an American Gastroenterological Association technical review on ZD, there is a consensus recommending this type of surgery[3].

The endoscopic treatment of ZD can achieve the same clinical results as surgical treatment while reducing the incidence of complications and mortality[4–7]. In 1917, Mosher described for the first time the endoscopic treatment of ZD, but this procedure was only disseminated by Dohlman and Mattson in the 1960s[8]. They developed a special rigid, double-lipped laryngoscope, and the ZD bridge was cut by using insulated forceps and a diathermic knife. Van Overbeek et al.[9] introduced the use of CO_2 laser applying a similar rigid laryngoscope. A variation of this approach is the stapler-assisted method. Endoscopic stapling oesophagodiverticulostomy has also been shown by Collard et al.[10] to be a safe and effective procedure, but always requiring general anaesthesia and a special long, rigid diverticuloscope, which is not suitable for patients with a small diverticulum. This procedure may also cause dental injuries in elderly patients with arthritis who are not able to overextend their neck.

The endoscopic intraluminal treatment of ZD by use of a flexible endoscope is nowadays an alternative to surgical treatment. A monopolar forceps or a needle knife is used to cut the ZD bridge. Argon plasma coagulation (APC) has also been used for this purpose. In order to have a better view during the procedure, devices were developed such as a hood attached to the endoscope[11] and a flexible overtube called a diverticuloscope[12]. The first human trials describing endoscopic myotomy through a flexible endoscope were published simultaneously by Ishioka et al. and Mulder et al.[4,5]. They used an electrocautery to incise the septum after placing a nasogastric tube for guidance. Primarily, the best indication for endoscopic therapy has been ZD in aged patients with comorbidities[4]. More than 90% of patients may have good relief of dysphagia, although 5–15% of patients will present recurrence due to the residual diverticulum and, in such cases, endoscopic retreatment may again be possible[13]. Cervical or mediastinal emphysema occurs in 0–23% of patients and bleeding in 0–10% of patients following endoscopic cricopharyngeal myotomy[14]. Mortality is usually caused by complications unrelated to the procedure[13].

The use of domestic pigs as an animal model for training ZD endoscopic treatment is well established and also helpful to the development of new techniques and accessories[15]. In our experimental laboratory the use of harmonic scissors through a flexible overtube allowed a quick and feasible procedure without bleeding, and with good visualization of the bottom of the diverticulum[16].

Therefore, the use of an animal model for training ZD endoscopic treatment is welcome and quite helpful, because it reproduces a similar situation to that found in humans. In addition, this animal model might be helpful in the further development of new ZD treatment techniques and accessories, such as the flexible stapler and the flexible harmonic scissor.

Part 1: References

1. Veenker EA, Andersen PE, Cohen JI. Cricopharyngeal spasm and Zenker's diverticulum. Head Neck. 2003;25:681–93.
2. Aggerholm K, Illum P. Surgical treatment of Zenker's diverticulum. J Laryngol Otol. 1990;104:312–14.
3. Cook IJ, Kahrilas PJ. AGA Technical review on the management of oropharyngeal dysphagia. Gastroenterology. 1999;116:455–78.
4. Ishioka S, Sakai P, Maluf Filho F, Melo JM. Endoscopic incision of Zenker's diverticula. Endoscopy. 1995;27:433–7.
5. Mulder CJ, den Hartog G, Robijn RJ, Thies JE. Flexible endoscopic treatment of Zenker's diverticulum: a new approach. Endoscopy. 1995;27:438–42.
6. Hashiba K, de Paula AL, da Silva JG et al. Endoscopic treatment of Zenker's diverticulum. Gastrointest Endosc. 1999;49:93–7.
7. Waye JD, Sakai P, Belsaguy AF, Devière J, Hassid S, Mulder CJ. Treatment of Zenker's diverticulum. Gastrointest Endosc. 2001;54:135–7.

8. Dohlman G, Mattson O. The endoscopic operation for hypopharyngeal diverticula: a roentgen-cinematographic study. AMA Arch Otolaryngol. 1960;71:744–52.
9. Van Overbeek JJ, Hoeksema PE, Edens ET. Microendoscopic surgery of the hypopharyngeal diverticulum using electrocoagulation or carbon dioxide laser. Ann Otol Rhinol Laryngol. 1984;93:34–6.
10. Collard JM, Otte JB, Kestens PJ. Endoscopic stapling technique of esophagodiverticulostomy for Zenker's diverticulum. Ann Thorac Surg. 1993;56:573–6.
11. Sakai P, Ishioka S, Maluf-Filho F, Chaves D, Moura EG. Endoscopic treatment of Zenker's diverticulum with an oblique-end hood attached to the endoscope. Gastrointest Endosc. 2001;54:760–3.
12. Evrard S, Le Moine O, Hassid S, Devière J. Zenker's diverticulum: a new endoscopic treatment with a soft diverticuloscope. Gastrointest Endosc. 2003;58:116–20.
13. Mulder CJ, Costamagna G, Sakai P. Zenker's diverticulum: treatment using a flexible endoscope. Endoscopy. 2001;33:991–7.
14. Ferreira LE, Simmons DT, Baron TH. Zenker's diverticula: pathophysiology, clinical presentation, and flexible endoscopic management. Dis Esophagus. 2008;21:1–8.
15. Seaman DL, de la Mora Levy J, Gostout CJ, Rajan E, Herman L, Knipschield M. An animal training model for endoscopic treatment of Zenker's diverticulum. Gastrointest Endosc. 2007;65:1050–3.
16. Hondo F, Maluf-Filho F, Nappi JG, Sakai P. Endoscopic diverticulotomy by harmonic scissor: an experimental model. Endoscopy. 2008 (In press).

PART 2: ENDOSCOPIC TREATMENT OF OESOPHAGEAL AND GASTRIC VARICES

OESOPHAGEAL VARICES SCREENING

Screening for oesophageal varices with upper gastrointestinal (GI) endoscopy (EGD) is recommended in patients with hepatic cirrhosis[1–3]. Capsule endoscopy (CE) is an alternative to EGD. In a multicentre study comparing EGD to CE, the latter was found to have an 84% sensitivity and 88% specificity in detecting oesophageal varices[4]. Although showing good tolerance and satisfaction, CE requires further studies to determine its accuracy in the detection of oesophageal varices, and may be an alternative to patients who are unable or refuse to undergo EGD.

PREVENTION OF THE FIRST VARICEAL BLEEDING (PRIMARY PROPHYLAXIS)

For patients with portal hypertension (hepatic venous pressure gradient (HVPG) >6 mmHg) and no oesophageal varices, the use of non-selective beta-blockers was not effective in the prevention of variceal development in addition to related side-effects. Therefore, its use in this situation is not recommended[5].

In patients with small varices and signs of high risk of bleeding (Child C and presence of red wale markings), beta-blockers should be recommended for preventing the first variceal haemorrhage and they may be used in patients not fulfilling criteria for increased risk of bleeding. In patients using non-selective beta-blockers an EGD follow-up is not necessary. For those who are not under this medication, EGD should be repeated within 2 years[6].

For patients with medium/large varices, two therapies are available: non-selective beta-blockers and endoscopic band ligation (EBL). The Baveno IV consensus recommends non-selective beta-blockers for primary prophylaxis, and EBL should be considered for patients with contraindications, intolerance or non-compliance with non-selective beta-blockers. EBL is associated with a small but significantly lower incidence of first variceal haemorrhage without differences in mortality. However, EBL long-term benefits are uncertain because of the short follow-up duration. The AASLD/ACG (American Association for the Study of Liver Diseases/American College of Gastroenterology) deems both treatments as efficient in the prevention of the first variceal bleeding in high risk of haemorrhage (Child B/C or variceal red wale markings on endoscopy) and considers that the therapeutic decision depends on the characteristics and preferences of patients, as well as local resources and experience. Although EBL is apparently related to fewer occurrences of first bleeding, non-selective beta-blockers also prevent other bleeding sources in portal hypertension, such as gastric varices and portal gastropathy, in addition to suggesting a possible reduction of spontaneous bacterial peritonitis. Studies on the combined use of EBL and non-selective beta-blockers were inconclusive and, given the unacceptable risk–benefit ratio, this approach cannot be currently recommended[6].

TREATMENT OF ACUTE VARICEAL BLEEDING

The treatment of acute variceal bleeding should at first take into account the protection of airways prior to endoscopy in order to prevent pulmonary aspiration, especially in patients with changes in consciousness level due to hepatic encephalopathy. Orotracheal intubation should also be taken into account for patients with uncontrollable bleeding.

Volaemic reposition should be immediately started to prevent complications such as hypovolaemic shock and renal failure. Antibiotics, such as quinolone and third-generation cephalosporin, should be administered to all patients for 5–7 days because they reduce mortality rates, infection risks and rebleeding rates. Vasoactive drugs (somatostatin or its analogues, octreotide and vapreotide, and terlipressin) should be administered at admission of a patient with suspect of variceal bleeding and kept for 2–5 days. Terlipressin is the drug of choice, with somatostatin and analogous drugs as second choice[7].

Endoscopic therapy is usually performed within the first 12 h. EBL has been considered as the first choice because this is an easier technique with fewer complications than sclerosis, requiring an experienced and skilled endoscopist. Some studies demonstrate that, in centres experienced in the use of sclerosis, results are found to be similar to those obtained with EBL in the control of acute variceal bleeding[8].

Failure to control bleeding or rebleeding may be treated again with endoscopic therapy. In selected patients especially those with HVPG >20 mmHg, the placement of a TIPS (transjugular intrahepatic portosystemic shunt) may be an acceptable option because studies point out a significant improvement in survival rates.

PREVENTION OF VARICEAL BLEEDING RECURRENCE (SECONDARY PROPHYLAXIS)

The best approach for patients with oesophageal varices with prior bleeding episode is the combined treatment of non-selective beta-blockers and EBL. Non-selective beta-blockers protect against bleeding before the eradication of varices with EBL, and also prevent the recurrence of varices after completing endoscopic treatment. The secondary prophylaxis with non-selective beta-blockers should be initiated when the patient has been haemodynamically stable. Endoscopic treatment may be started 1–2 weeks after the bleeding episode up to complete variceal eradication[3]. The first follow-up endoscopy may be performed within 1–3 months after the eradication and every 6–12 months after that. This initial follow-up should be very strict because of the high recurrence of varices within the first 2 years (approximately 50%).

Sclerotherapy is usually not indicated in secondary prophylaxis. Studies indicate a significantly lower risk of rebleeding with the use of EBL, and fewer sessions are necessary to eradicate varices. Furthermore, complications concerning sclerotherapy are more frequent and severe[9].

GASTRIC VARICES

There is less evidence concerning how to deal with gastric varices in comparison with oesophageal varices, due to few controlled studies[3]. Although gastric varices bleed less frequently than oesophageal varices, bleeding intensity and mortality rates are higher. Gastric varices occur in approximately 20% of patients with portal hypertension. Fundal varices (IGV1) are those with higher bleeding and rebleeding rates and non-selective beta-blockers are recommended as primary prophylaxis.

The pharmacological treatment for acute bleeding is similar to that for oesophageal variceal bleeding. In the initial endoscopic treatment, obliteration of varices with cyanoacrylate injection is recommended. TIPS should be taken into account for patients who do not respond to pharmacological and endoscopic treatments[6]. There is no consensus on primary prophylaxis of gastric varices.

Part 2: References

1. de Franchis R. Evolving consensus in portal hypertension. Report of the Baveno IV consensus workshop on methodology of diagnosis and therapy in portal hypertension. J Hepatol. 2005;43:167–76.
2. Garcia-Tsao G, Sanyal AJ, Grace ND, Carey WD. Prevention and management of gastroesophageal varices and variceal hemorrhage in cirrhosis. Am J Gastroenterol. 2007;102:2086–102.
3. Garcia-Tsao G, Sanyal AJ, Grace ND, Carey WD. Prevention and management of gastroesophageal varices and variceal hemorrhage in cirrhosis. Hepatology. 2007;46:922–38.
4. de Franchis R, Eisen GM, Eliakim AR et al. Esophageal capsule endoscopy (PillCam ESO) is comparable to traditional endoscopy for detection of esophageal varices. An international multi-center trial. Gastrointest Endosc. 2007;65:AB107.

5.   Groszmann RJ, Garcia-Tsao G, Bosch Jet al. Beta-blockers to prevent gastroesophageal varices in patients with cirrhosis. N Engl J Med. 2005;353:2254–61.
6.   Garcia-Tsao G, Bosch J, Groszmann RJ. Portal hypertension and variceal bleeding – unresolved issues. Summary of an American Association for the Study of Liver Diseases and European Association for the Study of the Liver single-topic conference. Hepatology. 2008;47:1764–72.
7.   Bendtsen F, Krag A, Moller S. Treatment of acute variceal bleeding. Dig Liver Dis. 2008;40:328–36.
8.   Boix J, Lorenzo-Zúñiga V, Moreno de Vega V, Domènech E, Gassull MA. Sclerotherapy and esophageal variceal bleeding: time to forget it, or not? Endoscopy. 2007;39:478.
9.   Kravetz D. Prevention of recurrent esophageal variceal hemorrhage: review and current recommendations. J Clin Gastroenterol. 2007;41:S318–22.

PART 3: PALLIATIVE TREATMENT FOR MALIGNANT OESOPHAGEAL OBSTRUCTION

INTRODUCTION

Palliative therapy for advancedoesophageal cancer is frequently necessary for patients with unresectable disease, poor medical condition or local recurrence[1].

Dysphagia, the most disabling symptom, is associated with increasing weight loss, local discomfort and aspiration pneumonia. Palliative resection is associated with a 20–60% morbidity and a 10–33% mortality. Symptoms only develop after 50% or more of the luminal diameter is involved, resulting in late presentation and poor prognosis (5-year survival of 5–10%)[2].

Median survival time for patients with inoperable disease is 4–6 months and rapid and lasting restoration of swallowing is the main goal of palliative treatment[3].

PALLIATIVE MODALITIES

Surgical bypass

Surgical bypass is advocated by some surgeons on the basis that it results in relief of dysphagia better than other palliative modalities. The mortality rate is 40% or higher and food intake is comparable to self-expandable metal stents (SEMS)[4,5].

Chemotherapy (CT) and radiotherapy (RT)

Chemotherapy has been used for metastatic oesophageal cancer, but current trials have failed to demonstrate improvement in survival[6]. Dysphagia relief achieved with combinations of cisplatin, epirubicin and 5-fluorouracyl (5-FU) is 59–89%, and agents such as paclitaxel, irinotecan and lobaplatin may improve rates further[7]. Local chemotherapy administration into the tumour to minimize toxicity is currently under evaluation with cisplatin/epinephrine gel injections[8].

Radiotherapy is divided into external beam radiotherapy (EBRT), brachytherapy and combination radiotherapy. EBRT regimens are based on 30–60 Gy in 10 or more fractions given over a 5–6-week period. Results in dysphagia relief are unpredictable at around 50%, many patients are also seen to relapse rapidly after treatment. Brachytherapy is replacing radiotherapy source close to the tumour, maximizing the dose while minimizing damage to local structures. Results for swallowing improvement are 61–67%. Like EBRT, the procedure is straightforward, quick and relatively inexpensive, and treatment may be given on an outpatient basis. Combination radiotherapy can improve dysphagia relief up to 90%.

Chemoradiation therapy (CT-RT) has an effect in local and systemic disease, as well as chemotherapeutic radiosensitization of tumour providing dysphagia relief with acceptable toxicity. Improvement in swallowing is 75–90%, and 60% of patients remain dysphagia-free until death. Median dysphagia-free duration is 5 months. Severe toxicity is 12–30% and mortality 2%[7,9].

Oesophagitis and fistula formation occur in 20–30% of patients and post-radiation stricture in 30–50% of patients[2]. Chemoradiation and radiotherapy do not improve dysphagia immediately, requiring a 4–6-week period, and thus is not suitable for patients with expected survival of less than 3 months or suspected tracheo-oesophageal fistula[10].

Dilation

Dilation may be used with expandable balloons or wire-guided polyvinyl bougies under fluoroscopic control, allowing consumption of a soft diet. Blind Maloney dilations are associated with perforation increase in complex strictures. Benefits are usually brief, requiring repeated dilations within 1–2 weeks. Dilation is usually performed prior to endoscopic assessment, ablation therapy, and placement of an enteral feeding tube[1,8].

Nd-YAG laser

The use of laser for obstructing oesophageal cancer is a type of thermal ablation. It is not useful for extrinsic compression but may be more appropriate for exophytic, straight, short (<5 cm), non-circumferential mid-oesophageal tumours. A high-power Nd-YAG laser provides dysphagia palliation by thermal necrosis and vaporization of malignant tissue with endoscopic control[1,2,7].

Tumour is usually ablated in a circumferential retrograde manner (distal to proximal) after previous dilation allowing treatment of longer lesions, greater improvement in dysphagia, and fewer treatment sessions[2]. In general, two to four sessions are required for initial dysphagia relief and further treatment every 4–8 weeks. Technical success may be as high as 90%, functional success rate 80%, morbidity 6.7%, and mortality 3.6%.

Disadvantages of laser ablation are equipment cost and availability, besides being technically demanding and time-consuming, requiring repeated treatment. As such, laser ablation is increasingly viewed as a complementary therapy to improve dysphagia before curative surgery, to deal with postoperative recurrence or to manage tumour overgrowth and ingrowth in stent patients[7,8].

Electrocautery

Monopolar and bipolar electrocautery are infrequently used, and have proven to be difficult to control. BICAP has a high perforation rate, needs prior dilation, requires several treatment sessions, and has a 360° dispersion of energy, and therefore may be used only in fully circumferential lesions.

Argon plasma coagulation is a type of monopolar diathermy electrocautery using ionized argon gas. Despite great similarity to, and having the same treatment indications as for laser, argon plasma coagulation provides lower cost, availability, ease of use, low morbidity, and short learning curve. With limited depth of penetration (2–3 mm), it is also time-consuming and requires repeated treatment[2,7].

Injection therapy

Ethanol-induced tumour necrosis (ETN) is the least expensive endoscopic technique. Aliquots of 0.5–1 ml of 100% ethanol are injected into all visible tumour tissue (mean 8–10 ml per session), resulting in dysphagia relief within a week. Chest pain after treatment is common. If necessary, therapy may be repeated in 3–7 days; it is suitable for small localized exophytic and cervical tumours if a reasonable view is possible. Repeated treatment is often necessary and the pattern of tumour necrosis is unpredictable[2,7].

Photodynamic therapy (PDT)

Photodynamic therapy involves the interaction of a photosensitizing agent that preferentially concentrates in tumour tissue in combination with endoscopic low-power laser monochrome light (630 nm) exposure. The photochemical reaction in the presence of molecular oxygen produces cytotoxic, oxygen free radicals that cause microvessel damage, tissue ischaemia and necrosis[7,8].

Depth of penetration is about 5 mm and palliation is comparable to that achieved with Nd-YAG laser, but the procedure is easier to carry out and more comfortable for patients. PDT tends to provide better response for long (>8 cm) tumours and fewer perforation complications compared to laser (1% vs 7%)[7].

The major problem is light-sensitive drug retention in the skin for about 6–8 weeks after injection, and the need to avoid direct sun exposure during this period of time at risk of severe sunburn. Sunscreens are ineffective since they do not block visible light. Other drawbacks are the inability to relieve extrinsic compression, the frequent need for repeated treatment within 4–6 weeks, and considerable expense associated with the treatment[2,7,8]. A non-laser (Versa-light – ESC Medical Systems Ltd, Yokneam, Israel) has been applied as a monochromatic light source and was found to be less expensive and easier to move between hospital locations, besides being feasible and safe[11].

Endoprotheses and self-expanding metal stents (SEMS)

The advantages of endoscopic stent placement in malignant oesophageal obstruction are instant dysphagia relief, management of tracheo-oesophageal fistulas, and its applicability to both oesophageal cancer and mediastinal compression[12,13].

Stent placement technical success is 95–100% and functional success over 83–100%. Procedure-related perforations may occur in 4–7% of patients, chest pain in 10–60%, tumour overgrowth in 6–8.5%, late migration in 10–27%, and mortality in 0–8.5% owing to aspiration, perforation and haemorrhage[7].

Covered stents are the treatment of choice for managing tracheo-oesophageal fistulas, and successful palliation has been achieved in 70–80% of cases, although fistula enlargement or further fistula formation may occur. Patients with associated tracheobronchial stenosis must have respiratory stenosis treated first[1,13].

Tumours located in the cervical segment are difficult to manage due to intolerable foreign-body sensation, risk of perforation and migration to hypopharynx. Stenting of the distal oesophagus and gastric cardia also constitute a particular problem due to gastro-oesophageal reflux with a 3–9% aspiration risk[7,14]. In comparison with stents placed in more proximally located oesophageal tumours, palliation is inferior and may have a higher complication rate. Specially designed stents for cervical segment and SEMS with antireflux valve are available to be placed at these locations[15–17].

Prior or subsequent radiation and/or chemotherapy may increase the risk of stent-related complications. However, this relationship is still controversial and is currently under evaluation[14].

Expandable plastic stents were developed to offer an easier insertion with some decrease in cost[1,2]. A comparative study with self-expandable plastic stents and self-expandable metal stents demonstrated similar immediate results, and late obstruction occurred more often in the metal type[12].

Semi-rigid plastic tubes are less expensive, but their insertion procedure is traumatic and associated with high rates of acute complications (5–15%) and mortality (2–4%)[1,2,12,13]. Despite an immediate improvement in dysphagia, the need for additional interventions is frequent because of higher complication rates, and some authors advocate the use of chemoradiation as first-line palliative therapy for malignant oesophageal obstruction[18].

CONCLUSIONS

Chemoradiation and brachytherapy appear to be the first-line therapy for patients with malignant oesophageal obstruction with longer estimated survival rate (6 months or more), because of the long-term better quality of life and longer dysphagia-free period. SEMS is suitable for patients who failed to improve or presented recurrence after CT and/or RT treatment, when tracheo-oesophageal fistulas are present and in patients with an estimated survival rate of 3–4 months. Patients with very short life expectancy (few days) do not benefit from most of the palliative procedures, and less invasive methods should be offered, such as feeding tubes[19].

Part 3: References

1. Lightdale CJ. Esophageal cancer: practice guidelines. Am J Gastroenterol. 1999;94:20–9.
2. Kubba AK, Krasner N. An update in the palliative management of malignant dysphagia. Eur J Surg Oncol. 2000;26:116–29.
3. O'Hanlon DM, Callanan K, Karat D, Crisp W, Griffin SM. Outcome, survival, and costs in patients undergoing intubation for carcinoma of the esophagus. Am J Surg. 1997;174:316–19.
4. Watson A. Diagnosis and therapy for advanced esophageal cancer. Curr Opin Gastroenterol. 2003;19:400–5.
5. Aoki T, Osaka Y, Takagi Y et al. Comparative study of self-expandable metallic stent and bypass surgery for inoperable esophageal cancer. Dis Esophagus. 2001;14:208–11.
6. Richel DJ, Vervenne WL. Systemic treatment of oesophageal cancer. Eur J Gastroenterol Hepatol. 2004;16:249–54.
7. Shenfine J, McNamee P, Steen N, Bond J, Griffin SM. A pragmatic randomised controlled trial of the cost-effectiveness of palliative therapies for patients with inoperable oesophageal cancer. Health Technol Assess. 2005;9:1–121.
8. Javle M, Ailawadhi S, Yang GY, Nwogu CE, Schiff MD, Nava HR. Palliation of malignant dysphagia in esophageal cancer: a literature-based review. J Support Oncol. 2006;4:365–79.
9. Lee SH. The role of oesophageal stenting in the non-surgical management of oesophageal strictures. Br J Radiol. 2001;74:891–900.
10. Harvey JA, Bessell JR, Beller E et al. Chemoradiation therapy is effective for the palliative treatment of malignant dysphagia. Dis Esophagus. 2004;17:260–5.
11. Kashtan H, Konikoff F, Haddad R, Skornick Y. Photodynamic therapy of cancer of the esophagus using systemic aminolevulinic acid and a non laser light source: a phase I/II study. Gastrointest Endosc. 1999;49:760–4.
12. Dormann AJ, Eisendrath P, Wigginghaus B, Huchzermeyer H, Devière J. Palliation of esophageal carcinoma with a new self-expanding plastic stent. Endoscopy. 2003;35:207–11.
13. Sumiyoshi T, Gotoda T, Muro K et al. Morbidity and mortality after self-expandable metallic stent placement in patients with progressive or recurrent esophageal cancer after chemoradiotherapy. Gastrointest Endosc. 2003;57:882–5.
14. Leiper K, Morris AI. Treatment of oesophago-gastric tumours. Endoscopy. 2002;34:139–45.
15. Fontana MG, La Pinta ML, Moneghini D et al. Prognostic value of Goseki histological classification in adenocarcinoma of the cardia. Br J Cancer. 2003;88:401–5.
16. Laasch HU, Marriott A, Wilbraham L, Tunnah S, England RE, Martin DF. Effectiveness of open versus antireflux stents for palliation of the distal esophageal carcinoma and prevention of symptomatic gastroesophageal reflux. Radiology. 2002;225:359–65.
17. Shim CS, Jung IS, Bhandari S et al. Management of malignant strictures of the cervical esophagus with a newly-designed self-expanding metal stent. Endoscopy. 2004;36:554–7.
18. Ross WA, Alkassab F, Lynch PM et al. Evolving role of self-expanding metal stents in the treatment of malignant dysphagia and fistulas. Gastrointest Endosc. 2007;65:70–6.
19. Yajima K, Kanda T, Nakagawa S et al. Self-expandable metallic stents for palliation of malignant esophageal obstruction: special reference to quality of life and survival of patients. Dis Esophagus. 2004;17:71–5.

PART 4: ENDOSCOPIC TREATMENT OF GASTRO-OESOPHAGEAL REFLUX DISEASE

Gastro-oesophageal reflux disease (GORD) is one of the most common gastrointestinal disorders and, in the past decade, several endoluminal procedures for its treatment have been introduced. The purpose of endoscopic treatment is to obviate the need for long-term proton pump inhibitor (PPI) treatment and the potential morbidity of surgical or laparoscopic fundoplication. Endoscopic treatment can be divided into the following procedures:

- Endoscopic suturing and plication (Bard EndoCinch[®] and Wilson-Cook ESD – Endoscopic Suturing Device[®]) and full-thickness plication (NDO Plicator[®]).

- Thermal coagulation with radiofrequency device (Stretta[®]).

- Injection or implant of biopolymers into the gastro-oesophageal junction (Enteryx[®] and Gatekeeper[®]).

- Emerging techniques: endoscopic fundoplications (Esophyx[®], Hiz-Wiz[®], MediGus SRS[®], and Syntheon ARD[®]).

ENDOLUMENAL SUTURING AND PLICATION

The EndoCinch[®] (Bard Inc., Billerica, MA, USA) device was brought to commercial market in April 2000 for use as an endoscopic antireflux treatment. The procedure consists of two or three plications 1–2 cm below the gastro-oesophageal junction, under deep or conscious sedation. Clinical evidence has suggested that the plication is mostly anchored by the mucosal layer. The result is thus a weak valve that fails with pressure over time because of loss of sutures[1]. Subjective improvement, such as reduction of PPI and GORD scores, has been the main endpoint. Objective parameters, such as pH study, manometry and endoscopy, are not always considered. Uncontrolled short-term follow-up studies demonstrated a therapeutic benefit mainly considering the clinical parameter[2]. Unfortunately, follow-up periods ranging from 12 to 24 months after an EndoCinch[®] procedure have shown the lack of sustained response, meaning unsatisfactory results[3]. According to the manufacturer, over 4000 patients were treated using the EndoCinch[®] device for antireflux purpose. This device is still being manufactured and some investigators are using it for the endoscopic treatment of obesity.

ESD[®] (Endoscopic Suturing Device, Wilson-Cook Medical Inc., Winston-Salem, NC, USA), similar to the EndoCinch[®] device, does not require an overtube and easily applies sutures. However, sutures created partial-thickness plication and were not effective. In 2004, owing to unsuccessful results, the manufacturer withdrew the ESD[®] device from the market.

The NDO Plicator[®] (NDO Surgical Inc., Mansfield, MA, USA) device was designed to perform a full-thickness plication. The procedure consists of placing a single suture below the gastro-oesophageal junction in direct endoscopic visualization to create a full-thickness plication and a longer-lasting gastro-oesophageal valve. In a short- and long-term follow-up, clinical results were similar to those in previous publications evaluating the effect of EndoCinch[®][4]. Failure in clinical efficacy was attributable to the limitations of a single suture implant, which may be insufficient to create an effective antireflux barrier. In our personal (unpublished) study, we compared two small groups: one comprising 20 patients treated with single suture and another comprising 10 patients treated with double suture. No difference in clinical and objective parameters was found in either group after 12 months. In April 2008, the NDO Plicator® manufacturer ceased activities and this device is no longer available.

THERMAL COAGULATION – STRETTA® PROCEDURE

Radiofrequency energy has been applied for the treatment of disorders such as aberrant cardiac conduction pathways (Wolff–Parkinson–White syndrome), prostatic tumour and liver solid tumour. The Stretta® (Curon Medical Inc., Sunnyvale, CA, USA) device was approved for clinical use to treat GORD in 2000, and consists in the application of thermal radiofrequency at the level of the lower oesophageal sphincter (LOS) and gastric cardia. The device comprises a special balloon with multiple radially placed nickel–titanium needle electrodes. This device delivers controlled coagulation energy (80 V) achieving a target tissue temperature of 85°C for 2 min[5]. Data evaluating the clinical efficacy Stretta® vary across published studies, but surprisingly there are series of patients off PPI medication with sustained improvement in 75–86% at 48 months after the procedure[6,7]. Some authors have speculated that the denervation of sensitive nerve endings leads to a decrease in the perception of acid reflux and symptoms. Some patients who did not have oesophagitis before the procedure may develop this condition[8]. In November 2006, Curon Medical, the manufacturer of Stretta® went out of business; therefore this device is unavailable at the moment.

INJECTION/IMPLANT OF BIOPOLYMERS

Injection of Enteryx® (Boston Scientific Inc., Natick, MA, USA) into the muscle layer at the gastro-oesophageal junction for the treatment of GORD was approved in the United States in April 2003. The expected mechanism of action is the alteration in the gastro-oesophageal junction distensibility and configuration. Fibrous encapsulation might lengthen the LOS, potentially leading to an elevated threshold for LOS relaxation (LOSR)[9]. Clinical trials of an initial symptomatic multicentre study demonstrated the sustained effectiveness and safety of Enteryx® injections in PPI-dependent patients with GORD. At the 12-month evaluation, improvement in GORD health-related quality of life (GORD-HRQL) symptoms was verified in 78% of patients and in 73% of patients off PPI. At 24-month evaluation, 67% of patients eliminated the use of PPI and 72% reduced PPI dosage in 50% or greater[10]. Probably, due to the occurrence of complications with deaths, the manufacturer voluntarily withdrew this product from the market in September 2005.

The Gatekeeper® Reflux Repair System (Medtronic Inc., Minneapolis, MN, USA) is an expandable hydrogel pellet-like prosthesis, which is introduced into the distal oesophageal submucosa to augment the LOS[11]. In a European multicentre trial 40% of patients had achieved a normal pH level and median LOS pressure increased significantly, and 53% of patients were off PPI after 6 months. However, at 6 months only 70% of the prostheses were retained. This system was introduced for clinical use in the European Union in May 2003 and the company itself ceased to manufacture the device in October 2005.

EMERGING TECHNIQUES

Esophyx® (EndoGastric Solutions Inc., Redmond, WA, USA) is a new device developed for GORD treatment through an omega-shaped fundoplication. The technology is promising and preliminary clinical results in 19 patients with non-reducible hiatal hernia have shown significant improvement in the reduction of GORD symptoms, PPI use, hiatal hernia, and oesophagitis after 24 months[12]. Nevertheless, clinical evaluation based on a larger patient population is still to be assessed.

Other devices such as Hiz-Wiz®, MediGus SRS® and Syntheon ARD® are currently undergoing FDA review and no clinical trials are available.

DISCUSSION

In the past decade three different approaches to the endoscopic treatment of GORD have been developed: intraluminal endoscopic suturing and plication, radiofrequency thermal coagulation, and injection/implant of bulking agents into the lower oesophagus. In a short period of time six different devices and techniques were delivered to the market based on little preliminary data or safety and clinical efficacy. On the other hand, five of these six devices were removed from the market over this same period of time, and EndoCinch® is the only one to remain in use by some investigators for the endoscopic treatment of obesity[13]. Asymptomatic improvement has been shown for the majority of treated patients in short-term follow-up, but variable outcomes for the reduced need for PPI and pH studies have demonstrated the normalization of distal oesophageal acid exposure only for the minority. In all protocols, patients with significant reflux, oesophagitis, hiatal hernia more than 2 cm in size or Barrett's oesophagus are not typical candidates for this antireflux intervention. These considerations, in our own experience using four different techniques (EndoCinch®, ESD®, Enteryx®, and NDO Plicator®) reinforced the idea that those devices were not for routine use outside the research setting at Sao Paulo University Medical School. Two systematic reviews on this issue were recently published[8,14]. The authors of both reviews conclude that to date there are insufficient scientific and clinical data on safety, efficacy and durability to support the use of endoluminal therapies for GORD in routine clinical practice. Conceivably, some effective endoscopic technique might be available in the future, but no definite indication for endoscopic therapy of GORD is currently available. There are several newer devices under study or in development, and further testing and experience will demonstrate their capabilities in the treatment of GORD.

Part 4: References

1. Schiefke I, Zabel-Langhenning A, Neumann S, Feisthammel J, Moessner J, Caca K. Long term failure of endoscopic gastroplication (EndoCinch). Gut. 2005;54:752–8.
2. Filipi CJ, Lehman GA, Rothstein RI et al. Transoral, flexible endoscopic suturing for treatment of gastro-oesophageal reflux disease: a one year prospective follow up. Gut. 2003;52:34–9.
3. Abou-Rebyeh H, Hoepffner N, Rösch T et al. Long-term failure of endoscopic suturing in the treatment of gastroesophageal reflux: a prospective follow-up study. Endoscopy. 2005;37:213–16.
4. Pleskow D, Rothstein R, Kozarek R, Haber G, Gostout C, Lembo A. Endoscopic full-thickness plication for the treatment of GERD: long-term multicenter results. Surg Endosc. 2007;21:439–44.
5. Triadafilopoulos G. Changes in GERD symptom scores correlate with improvement in esophageal acid exposure after the Stretta procedure. Surg Endosc. 2004;18:1038–44.
6. Reymunde A, Santiago N. Long-term results of radiofrequency energy delivery for the treatment of GERD: sustained improvements in symptoms, quality of life, and drug use at 4-year follow-up. Gastrointest Endosc. 2007;65:361–6.
7. Noar MD, Lotfi-Emran S. Sustained improvement in symptoms of GERD and antisecretory drug use: 4-year follow-up of the Stretta procedure. Gastrointest Endosc. 2007;65:367–72.
8. Fry LC, Mönkemüller K, Malfertheiner P. Systematic review: Endoluminal therapy for gastro-oesophageal reflux disease: evidence from clinical trials. Eur J Gastroenterol Hepatol. 2007;19:1125–39.
9. Johnson DA, Ganz R, Aisenberg J et al. Endoscopic, implantation of enteryx for treatment of GERD: 12-month results of a prospective, multicenter trial. Am J Gastroenterol. 2003;98:1921–30.
10. Cohen LB, Johnson DA, Ganz RA et al. Enteryx implantation for GERD: expanded multicenter trial results and interim postapproval follow-up to 24 months. Gastrointenst Endosc. 2005;61:650–8.
11. Kahrilas PJ, Lee TJ. Gatekeeper reflux repair system: a mechanistic hypothesis. Gut. 2005;54:179–80.
12. Dapri G, Rajan A, Himpens J, Cadiere GB. Transoral incisionless fundoplication: results at 2 years. Gastrointest Endosc. 2008;67:AB138.
13. Fogel R, Raijman I, Frontera J, Bonilla Y, La Fuente RD. Comparison of continued versus interrupted suturing during endoscopic vertical gastroplasty in the management of morbid obesity. Gastrointest Endosc. 2007;65:AB280.
14. Pace F, Costamagna G, Penagini R, Repici A, Annese V. Review article: Endoscopic antireflux procedures – an unfulfilled promise? Aliment Pharmacol Ther. 2008;27:375–84.

2
Oesophagus: innovations

J. POHL

Barrett's oesophagus is the premalignant lesion for the majority of patients with oesophageal adenocarcinoma[1]. In order to detect neoplasias at early and curable stages endoscopic surveillance for patients with Barrett's oesophagus has been advocated[2-4]. High-grade intra-epithelial neoplasias (HGIN) and early cancer (EC) are often discrete or macroscopically occult lesions and therefore directed biopsies in combination with four-quadrant random biopsies according to the Seattle protocol are recommended as the gold standard for surveillance[2-4]. However, since endoscopic mucosa resection instead of surgical oesophageal resection is becoming the method of choice for mucosal neoplasias[5-7], exact localization of HGIN/EC within the Barrett's segment is of the utmost importance. As four-quadrant biopsies are not only time-consuming and expensive, but are also associated with a basic imprecision, efforts have been made to develop novel endoscopic imaging techniques that may improve the detection of early lesions in Barrett's oesophagus.

The high-resolution endoscopy technique with high-quality charge-coupled device chips has significantly improved the detection of subtle mucosal lesions that are not readily visible with standard techniques[8,9]. Although there are no large validation studies, there is accumulating evidence that mucosal imaging of Barrett's oesophagus can be further increased by conventional chromoendoscopy with methylene blue[10,11] or acetic acid[12-14]. In our unit we prefer chromoendoscopy with acetic acid, since acetic acid can be directly applied to the mucosa and immediately evaluated. Acetic acid is not actively absorbed, but it induces whitening of the tissue surface with accentuation of the mucosal pit pattern[15]. However, conventional chromoendoscopy still has some problems, such as difficulty in achieving complete and even coating of the mucosal surface with the dye, the extra cost of the equipment for dye spraying, and the extra time required to perform the procedure. Even more importantly, chromoendoscopy is not useful for imaging of the capillary patterns that might be important in the early diagnosis of cancer[16].

To resolve the problems of conventional chromoendoscopy, virtual chromoendoscopy image systems called narrow-band imaging (NBI)[17-19] and 'Fuji Intelligent Color Enhancement' (FICE) were proposed. These methods are based on the optical phenomenon that the depth of light penetration into tissues is dependent on the wavelength, with visible blue light (425 nm) penetrating only superficially and thus giving optimal mucosal surface imaging. As a consequence of these findings, the NBI system narrows the bandwidth by using optical filters within the light source of a video endoscope system. Although based on the same principle, FICE technology is not based on alterations but is operated with a computed algorithm in the processor. FICE takes an ordinary endoscopic image from the video processor and arithmetically processes the reflected photons to reconstitute virtual images by increasing the relative intensity of narrowed blue light to a maximum and decreasing narrowed red and green light to a minimum.

Modifications of spectral features by NBI and FICE emphasize the pit pattern contrast as well as the capillary pattern, and thus provide imaging features additional to those of both conventional endoscopy and chromoendoscopy[17–21]. In recent preliminary studies, FICE and NBI appeared to be equivalent to conventional chromoendoscopy with acetic acid[21] and indigocarmine[19], respectively, for detection of neoplastic lesions within Barrett's oesophagus.

Virtual chromoendoscopy might have some advantages over conventional chromoendoscopy: First, the virtual chromoendosopy mode can be conveniently applied by pressing a button at the grip of the endoscope. In contrast to conventional chromoendoscopy white-light endoscopy and virtual chromoendoscopy images can be compared by switching back and forth between modes. There is no need for dyes, spraying catheters, or extensive rinsing and aspiration. Secondly, vascular patterns are enhanced by NBI and FICE but not by chromoendoscopy. In this regard we postulate that careful endoscopic inspection that involves both white light and conventional or virtual chromoendoscopy, followed by targeted biopsy sampling, is the most important factor that may lead to the detection and precise localization of early mucosal lesions in the majority of patients with Barrett's oesophagus. Future studies will have to clarify whether this sophisticated approach has the potential to entirely replace the need for four-quadrant random biopsies.

Another novel endoscopic tool that has attracted much interest is confocal laser endomicroscopy that enables the endoscopist to perform *in vivo* histological examination of the gastrointestinal mucosa and might distinguish between neoplastic and non-neoplastic tissue during ongoing endoscopy. By using current endomicroscopy systems the mucosa can be analysed at a magnification of about $1000 \times$, and with a maximum penetration depth of the scanning laser light of up to 250 μm. Preliminary studies have shown that normal squamous epithelium and neoplastic squamous epithelium[22] and Barrett's mucosa and Barrett's neoplasia[23] can be differentiated reliably using endomicroscopy. However, larger studies are necessary to show the performance of the system in 'real-world' conditions.

Although controversial, endoscopic screening for the presence of Barrett's oesophagus for individuals at high risk has been recommended in order to reduce cancer-related deaths. While standard upper endoscopy is an invasive tool for screening, oesophageal capsule endoscopy is an exciting new technique that utilizes a dual-camera wireless capsule and offers an alternative approach for the visualization of the oesophageal mucosa without the need for sedation and without the discomfort and risks of conventional endoscopy. Two prospective, blinded clinical trials showed that the sensitivity and specificity for Barrett's oesophagus was 67% and 84%[24] and 77% and 85%[25], respectively; therefore, although capsule endoscopy proved save and convenient in these studies, at the present time it cannot be recommended as a primary screening tool for Barrett's oesophagus in patients with chronic reflux symptoms. However, technological advances (higher rate of image capture, better resolution, and broader area of visualization) and the validation of existing ingestion protocols may further improve its diagnostic accuracy.

New sophisticated endoscopic imaging techniques such as high-resolution endoscopy and conventional and virtual chromoendoscopy enable detection of neoplasia at very early stages. A known negligible risk of haematogenous dissemination and lymph node metastasis of mucosal neoplasias, as well as significant oesophagectomy-associated morbidity and mortality, have been the driving forces behind the development of local, minimally invasive endoscopic therapies in this patient population. Endoscopic resection is considered to be curative if the tumour is confined to the mucosa, and clear basal margins of all resected mucosal specimens are confirmed histologically. Our group recently published the first prospective study providing long-term post-endoscopic mucosal resection (EMR) follow-up in patients with low-risk early Barrett's carcinoma[26]. In 100 patients with 144 resections with the 'suck-and-cut' technique there were no major complications, and 99% of patients achieved complete remission. Although these data show excellent success rates, conclusive evidence of superiority of local endoscopic therapy might be provided only by a randomized prospective clinical trial comparing endoscopic therapy with the surgical approach. Facing the excellent results of non-invasive endoscopic therapy this trial would be ethically doubtful and will probably never be conducted.

However, a recent retrospective cohort study by Prasad and colleagues[27] compared overall survival, rates of morbidity and mortality in 199 patients with high-grade Barrett's neoplasias treated endoscopically versus with oesophagectomy; 129 were treated with photodynamic therapy (PDT) (with or without EMR), and 70 were treated with oesophagectomy. In the PDT/EMR group stricture formation occurred in 35 patients and required dilation, and one perforation occurred following dilation and required subsequent partial oesophagectomy. During a 5-year follow-up, eight patients (6.2%) from the PDT cohort developed oesophageal adenocarcinoma (OAC) and were treated with either oesophagectomy or EMR, depending on the extent of cancer. None of these patients had metastatic disease and all were alive at the end of the follow-up. In the oesophagectomy cohort mortality was 1.4%, postoperative morbidity was 38%. The overall mortality was 9% over a median period of 57.4 months in the PDT group and 8.5% over 63.4 months in the oesophagectomy group. None of the treated patients died from OAC.

Taken together recent years have provided a considerable increase in the number of high-quality clinical trials that demonstrate the benefits of novel endoscopic imaging techniques when compared with standard endoscopy for detection of oesophageal neoplasias. FICE and NBI appear to be exciting additions to the diagnostic armentarium, allowing detailed evaluation of superficial vascular patterns; however, large, randomized, prospective clinical trials are needed to validate its diagnostic role in this patient population. Although promising, at the present time capsule endoscopy cannot be recommended as a primary screening tool for Barrett's oesophagus in patients with chronic gastro-oesophageal reflux because sensitivity for Barrett's mucosa is suboptimal. Accumulating data on long-tem outcomes for endoscopic treatment of mucosal Barrett's carcinoma demonstrate that alternative endoscopic therapies are not only safe, but as efficacious as the traditional surgical approach. Especially at high-volume centres these techniques have already replaced oesophagectomy. The combination of novel endoscopic techniques, diagnostic and therapeutic, will provide the endoscopist with much-needed tools that can considerably enhance the diagnosis and treatment of reflux disease, Barrett's oesophagus, and early oesophageal cancer.

References

1. Haggitt RC, Tryzelaar J, Ellis FH et al. Adenocarcinoma complicating columnar epithelium-lined (Barrett's) esaphagus. Am J Clin Pathol. 1978;70:1–5.
2. Corley DA, Levin TR, Habel LA et al. Surveillance and survival in Barrett's adenocarcinomas: a population-based study. Gastroenterology. 2002;122:633–40.
3. Sampliner RE. Updated guidelines for the diagnosis. surveillance, and therapy of Barrett's esophagus. Am J Gastroenterol. 2002;97:1888–95.
4. Levine DS, Haggitt RC, Blount PL et al. An endoscopic biopsy protocol can differentiate high-grade dysplasia from early adenocarcinoma in Barrett's esophagus. Gastroenterology. 1993;104:40–50.
5. Ell C, May A, Gossner L et al. Endoscopic mucosal resection of early cancer and high grade dysplasia in Barrett's esophagus. Gastroenterology. 2000;118:670–7.
6. Ell C, May A, Pech O et al. Curative endoscopic resection of early esophageal adenocarcinomas (Barrett's cancer). Gastrointest Endosc. 2007;65:3–10.
7. Peters FP, Kara MA, Rosmolen WD et al. Endoscopic treatment of high-grade dysplasia and early stage cancer in Barrett's esophagus. Gastrointest Endosc. 2005;61:506–14.
8. Guelrud M, Herrera I, Essenfeld H et al. Enhanced magnification endoscopy: a new technique to identify specialized intestinal metaplasia in Barrett's esophagus. Gastrointest Endosc. 2001;53:559–65.
9. Sharma P, Weston AP, Topalovski M et al. Magnification chromoendoscopy for the detection of intestinal metaplasia and dysplasia in Barrett's oesophagus. Gut. 2003;52:24–7.
10. Gossner L, Pech O, May A et al. Comparison of methylene blue-directed biopsies and four-quadrant biopsies in the detection of high-grade intraepithelial neoplasia and early cancer in Barrett's esophagus. Dig Liver Dis. 2006;38:724–9.
11. Canto MI, Yoshida T, Gossner L. Chromoendoscopy of intestinal metaplasia in Barrett's esophagus. Endoscopy. 2002;34:330–6.
12. Hoffman A, Kiesslich R, Bender A et al. Acetic acid-guided biopsies after magnifying endoscopy compared with random biopsies in the detection of Barrett's esophagus: a prospective randomized trial with crossover design. Gastrointest Endosc. 2006;64:1–8.
13. Guelrud M, Ehrlich EE. Endoscopic classification of Barrett's esophagus. Gastrointest Endosc. 2004;59:58–65.
14. Rey JF, Inoue H, Guelrud M. Magnification endoscopy with acetic acid for Barrett's esophagus. Endoscopy. 2005;37:583–6.
15. Lambert R, Rey JF, Sankaranarayanan R. Magnification and chromoscopy with the acetic acid test. Endoscopy. 2003;35:437–45.
16. Yagi K, Nakamura A, Sekine A. Comparison between magnifying endoscopy and histological, culture and urease test findings from the gastric mucosa of the corpus. Endoscopy. 2002;34:376–81.

17. Gono K, Yamazaki K, Doguchi N et al. Endoscopic observation of tissue by narrow-band illumination. Opt Rev. 2003;10:1–5.
18. Machida H, Sano Y, Hamamoto Y et al. Narrow-band imaging in the diagnosis of colorectal mucosal lesions: a pilot study. Endoscopy. 2004;36:1094–8.
19. Kara MA, Peters FP, Rosmolen WD et al. High-resolution endoscopy plus chromoendoscopy or narrow-band imaging in Barrett's esophagus: a prospective randomized crossover study. Endoscopy. 2005;37:929–36.
20. Pohl J, May A, Rabenstein T et al. Comparison of computed virtual chromoendoscopy and conventional chromoendoscopy with acetic acid for detection of neoplasia in Barrett's esophagus. Endoscopy. 2007;39:594–8.
21. Pohl J, May, A, Rabenstein T et al. Computed virtual chromoendoscopy: a new tool for enhancing tissue surface structures. Endoscopy. 2007;39:80–3.
22. Pech O, Rabenstein T, Manner H et al. Confocal laser endomicroscopy for *in vivo* diagnosis of early squamous cell carcinoma in the esophagus. Clin Gastroenterol Hepatol. 2009;6:89–94.
23. Kiesslich R, Gossner L, Goetz M et al. *In vivo* histology of Barrett's esophagus and associated neoplasia by confocal laser endomicroscopy. Clin Gastroenterol Hepatol. 2006;4:979–87.
24. Lin OS, Schembre DB, Mergener K et al. Blinded comparison of esophageal capsule endoscopy versus conventional endoscopy for diagnosis of Barrett's esophagus in patients with chronic gastroesophageal reflux. Gastrointest Endosc. 2007;65:577–83.
25. Sharma P, Wani S, Rastogi A et al. The diagnostic accuracy of esophageal capsule endoscopy in patients with gastroesophageal reflux disease and Barrett's esophagus: a blinded, prospective study. Am J Gastroenterol. 2008;103:525–32.
26. Ell C, May A, Pech O et al. Curative endoscopic resection of early esophageal adenocarcinomas (Barrett's cancer). Gastrointest Endosc. 2007;65:3–11.
27. Prasad GA, Wang KK, Buttar NE et al. Long-term survival following endoscopic and surgical management of high-grade dysplasia in Barrett's esophagus. Gastroenterology. 2007;132:1226–33.

7
Innovations in endoscopic ultrasound

P. VILMANN and V. SHARMA

INTRODUCTION

Endoscopic ultrasound (EUS) combines two modalities: endoscopic visualization and high-frequency ultrasound, thereby permitting precise delineation of the individual layers of the gastrointestinal tract as well as adjacent surrounding structures and organs. Ever since the introduction of endosonography in the early 1980s the method has undergone immense development, leading to an important method for clinical decision-making in a variety of indications in gastroenterology, pulmonal medicine and oncology[1-4]. This development, leading to what EUS is today, are mainly due to innovations that are developed during different time periods and may as such be regarded in different phases.

The aim of this chapter is to highlight innovations important to the present status of EUS and to look into future perspectives of EUS imaging and interventions.

HISTORY OF EUS INNOVATIONS

The innovations of EUS can be regarded in three important steps, i.e. first development of EUS imaging with radial mechanical transducers, secondly development of linear electronic transducer technology and finally development of EUS-guided intervention, including biopsy and therapeutic procedures (Table 1).

From 1980 to 1986 developments of endoscopes and miniprobes with mechanical transducers was initiated mainly by the Olympus company. Based on these developments numerous basic studies with delineation of the wall layers both under normal as well as abnormal conditions were published, and graduately indications for endosonography were established (Figure 1)[5,6].

During the period 1986-1991 the indications of EUS imaging with mechanical radial scanning transducers were established, including staging and evaluation of resectability of gastrointestinal (GI) cancer and GI lymphoma, evaluation of GI tract pathology (large gastric folds, submucosal tumours, impressions, vascular malformations etc.), evaluation of extrahepatic

Section II
Stomach

Chair: D COUMAROS, A REPICI and T TOYONAGA

Figure 2 The first curved linear array endoscope first used by the author in 1988 (Hitachi/Pentax, EC 124)

obstruction, diagnosis of common bile duct stones and microlithiasis, evaluation of pancreatitis, detection of neuroendocrine tumours and evaluation of cystic pancreatic tumours[2–8].

The next important step was development of an endoscope with a curved linear electronic transducer. The first prototype that was really considered of value for human use was developed in 1988 by Hitachi/Pentax (EC 124) and first used by our group[9] (Figure 2). However, it soon became clear that a biopsy channel was needed.

Based on these experiences another echoendoscope with a 2 mm biopsy channel was developed (Pentax/Hitachi, FG-32 UA) (Figure 3). This endoscope was used by our group in 1991.

From 1991 to 2000 further development of electronic transducer technology and EUS-FNA (fine needle aspiration) was done. Early needle testing for EUS-FNA was started by our group in 1991 in collaboration with Wilson Cook, Denmark, and the first EUS-guided FNA biopsy of a pancreatic lesion was performed in the same year (Figure 4)[10]. The first dedicated handle device with needle was created by our group during the period between 1991 and 1993 (Hancke/Vilmann needle, GIP/Medi-Globe, Achenmühle, Germany) (Figure 5)[11]. Gradually a variety of FNA needles with different diameters were developed by different companies from 1995 to 2008. All these devices were basicly similar to the original needle design.

Based on experiences from the late 1990s we realized the great potential of EUS-guided intervention. It became more and more clear that it was possible to reach regions in the human body that can either not be reached by other imaging modalities or are too minute to targeted (transcutaneously).

3
Stomach: innovations – endoscopic diagnosis and treatment of early gastric cancer

H. YAMAMOTO

INTRODUCTION

Complete cure of gastric cancer with non-resective therapy alone, including chemotherapy, remains difficult despite significant progress in medicine. However, complete cure of gastric cancer can be expected if lesions can be completely removed surgically. Therefore, early detection and early resection is still the best therapeutic strategy for gastric cancer. Recent innovations in endoscopic technology such as the high-definition endoscope, magnifying endoscope, narrow-band imaging (NBI), Fuji Intelligent Color Enhancement (FICE), endocytoscopy, and confocal laser endomicroscopy are promising advancements that can facilitate early detection of early gastric cancer (EGC). EGC is defined as a gastric carcinoma confined to the mucosa or submucosa, regardless of the presence or absence of regional lymph node metastases. The outcome of surgical therapy for EGC has been favourable, with a 5-year survival rate reaching 90–100% in Japan[1,2]. When endoscopic therapy is chosen for EGC because of its low invasiveness, complete cure should still be the goal, as it is for surgical treatment. The indications for endoscopic therapy thus need to be determined based on evaluation of curability. A recent innovation in endoscopic therapeutic technique, endoscopic submucosal dissection (ESD), has enabled reliable, complete en-bloc resection of ECG and enables detailed histopathological evaluation of whether treatment is curative[3].

INDICATIONS FOR USE OF ENDOSCOPIC THERAPY FOR EGC

Endoscopic treatment for EGC is beneficial because of its low invasiveness. However, it is important to note that complete curability should not be compromised by choice of less invasive therapy. Careful decisions regarding whether the indications for endoscopic therapy have been met are thus indispensable. In addition, detailed pathological examination of resected tissues enables precise determination as to whether cancers have been completely resected, allowing correct decisions regarding the need for additional surgery. The most important factor influencing the survival of patients with EGC is the presence or absence of lymph node metastasis[4-6]. The incidence of lymph node metastasis has been reported to be 1–3% for mucosal cancers and 11–20% for submucosal cancers of the stomach[5]. Lymph node dissection is beyond the capability of endoscopic therapy. Endoscopic therapy should thus be performed for EGC only when the risk of lymph node metastasis is negligible and cure is expected with complete local resection.

Based on the reports by Gotoda et al. at the National Cancer Center and other groups[7], the indications for ESD in Japan at the present time are considered to be as follows:

1. Non-ulcerated, differentiated-type mucosal carcinomas regardless of tumour size.

2. Differentiated-type mucosal carcinomas with an ulcer scar measuring 30 mm or less.

Lesions meeting the above criteria should be resected endoscopically in one piece. Resected tissues are sectioned at 2 mm intervals and submitted for pathological evaluation. Treatment can be considered curative when a differentiated-type mucosal carcinoma without submucosal invasion or lymphatic or venous invasion is completely resected with margins free of tumour.

ENDOSCOPIC DIAGNOSIS OF EGC

Detection of EGC

Early detection and accurate diagnosis are essential for successful endoscopic treatment of EGC.

Macroscopic types of gastric cancer, according to the Japanese Classification of Gastric Carcinoma, 2nd English edition, by the Japanese Gastric Cancer Association, are indicated in Table 1[8]. By macroscopic type, EGC are of type 0 morphology with a subclassification of type 0, as indicated in Figure 1. Type 0-IIa and 0-IIc, which are the superficial elevated type and superficial depressed type, are common morphologies of EGC. Because most EGC are superficial, the finding of modest changes in morphology and colour of the mucosa is important for their detection. The morphological characteristics of EGC include mild elevation and shallow depression of the mucosa, as well as discontinuity with surrounding mucosa and areas with uneven surface. For changes in colour, pale redness or fading is important[9].

However, these changes are so subtle that detection of EGC has been challenging with conventional endoscopic observation. Chromoendoscopy with indigo carmine spray can be used to enhance fine structure and colour contrast, resulting in improved accuracy of diagnosis (Figure 2)[10].

Table 1 Macroscopic types of gastric cancer

Type 0: Superficial, flat tumours with or without minimal elevation or depression 　　　Type 0-I: Protruded type 　　　Type 0-IIa: Superficial elevated type 　　　Type 0-IIb: Flat type 　　　Type 0-IIc: Superficial depressed type 　　　Type 0-III: Excavated type
Type 1: Polypoid tumours, sharply demarcated from the surrounding mucosa, usually attached on a wide base margin
Type 2: Ulcerated carcinomas with sharply demarcated and raised margins
Type 3: Ulcerated carcinomas without definite limits, infiltrating into the surrounding wall
Type 4: Diffusely infiltrating carcinomas in which ulceration is usually not a marked feature
Type 5: Non-classifiable carcinomas that cannot be classified into any of the above types

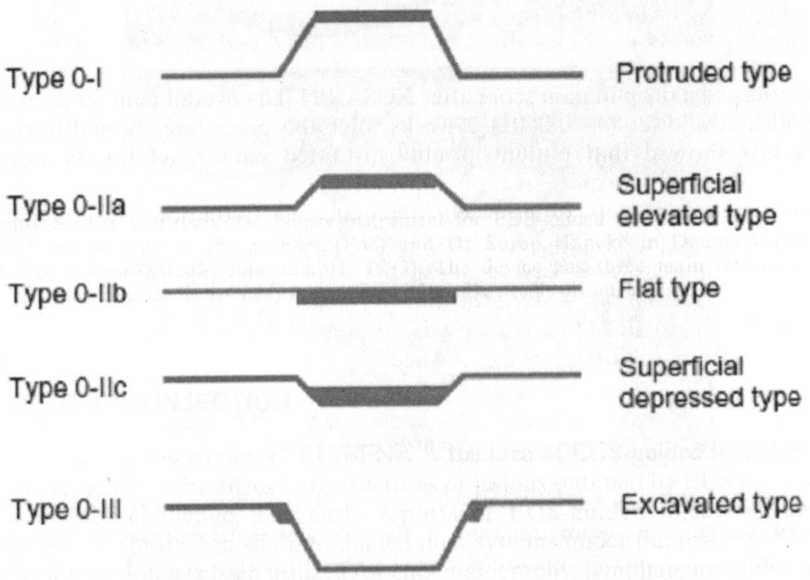

Figure 1 Subtypes of type 0 morphology. In the combined superficial types, the type occupying the largest area should be described first, followed by the next type, e.g. IIc + III. Types 0-I and 0-IIa are distinguished as follows: type 0-I, the lesion has a thickness of more than twice that of the normal mucosa; type 0-IIa, the lesion has a thickness up to twice that of the normal mucosa

NBI and FICE are recently developed technologies for optimizing visualization of subtle changes in lesions. Both NBI and FICE have a possibility of increasing detection rates by enhancing image contrast without use of dye spraying. Both systems can also be used for detailed examination with enhancement of vascular pattern combined with magnification.

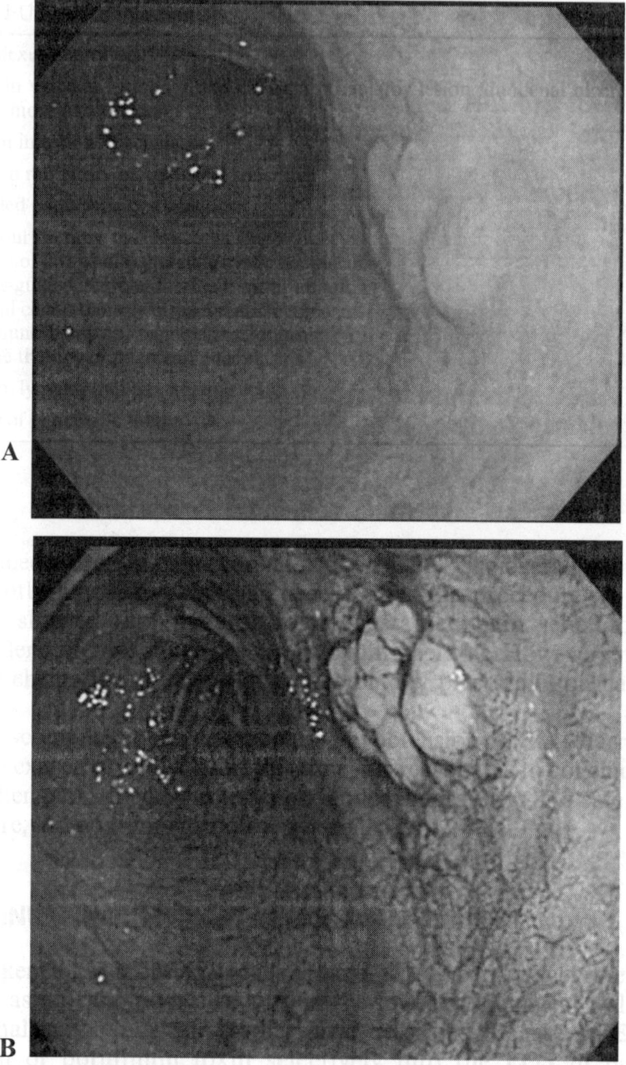

Figure 2   EGC, type 0-IIa, well-differentiated tubular adenocarcinoma (tub1), m, ly0, v0.
A: Conventional endoscopic image; **B**: chromoendoscopy with indigo carmine spray

NBI is a special imaging technique that uses spectral narrow-band optical filters that allow passage only of those spectral components of light (e.g. blue, 390–445 nm; green, 530–550 nm) that will be absorbed by haemoglobin in the mucosal blood vessels. The surrounding mucosa does not absorb, and instead reflects, most portions of this light and, because of this, maximum contrast of vessels and surrounding mucosa is achieved[11].

Because of the excellent enhancement of mucosal blood vessels afforded with this technique, the fine vascular pattern of the mucosal surface can be clearly observed. This is most useful for detailed examination combined with magnification[12].

However, improvement by NBI of detection rates has not been demonstrated in previous studies[13–15]. NBI is not optimal for detection, probably because distant views with it are too dark and no colour contrast is obtained between EGC and surrounding mucosa.

FICE is also termed optimal band imaging (OBI). With this system the spectral image for each wavelength is produced through the reflectance spectrum estimation technique from the white-light image. Three spectral images are selected and allocated to red–green–blue television signals for reconstruction of images[16].

With the FICE system, optimal wavelength bands can be chosen for the spectral images in accordance with the purpose of examination. By choosing optimal bands and adjusting the gain for allocated images, colour enhancement of lesions can be achieved. Using the FICE system, not only the vascular pattern but also the fine structural pattern of the mucosal surface can be enhanced. Because FICE provides bright images with a distant view without magnification, and colour contrast can be obtained between EGC and surrounding mucosa (Figure 3A,B), it is believed to have good potential for increasing the rate of detection of EGC[16]. Using FICE with a magnifying endoscope, detailed examination with enhancement of vascular pattern combined with magnification can be performed immediately after detection of a lesion (Figure 3C).

After endoscopic detection of EGC, it is confirmed histopathologically by taking biopsies. However, recent innovations in endoscopic technology might make biopsy unnecessary for confirmation. Endocytoscopy and confocal laser endomicroscopy are two promising technologies enabling instant magnification at the microscopic level. Using them, confirmation of EGC can be immediately performed at the time of detection of the lesion, facilitating endoscopic detection of EGC.

Following detection of EGC, determination of the depth of invasion and the extent of tumour is important for successful endoscopic treatment. The following are practical methods for this.

Determination of depth of invasion

Since the depth of invasion of EGC is strongly correlated with lymph node metastasis, pretreatment depth staging is important. Conventional endoscopy and endoscopic ultrasonography (EUS) have been shown to be useful for such staging.

It has been reported that depth staging based on conventional endoscopy has 70–80% accuracy. EGC of small protruded type (type 0-I) or superficial elevated type (type 0-IIa) with a smooth surface suggests mucosal cancer. Lesions with small shallow depressions, but without bank formation or uneven surfaces, are also indicative of mucosal cancer. Lesions with a more rigid base with an irregularly shaped nodule on the margin or folds that are

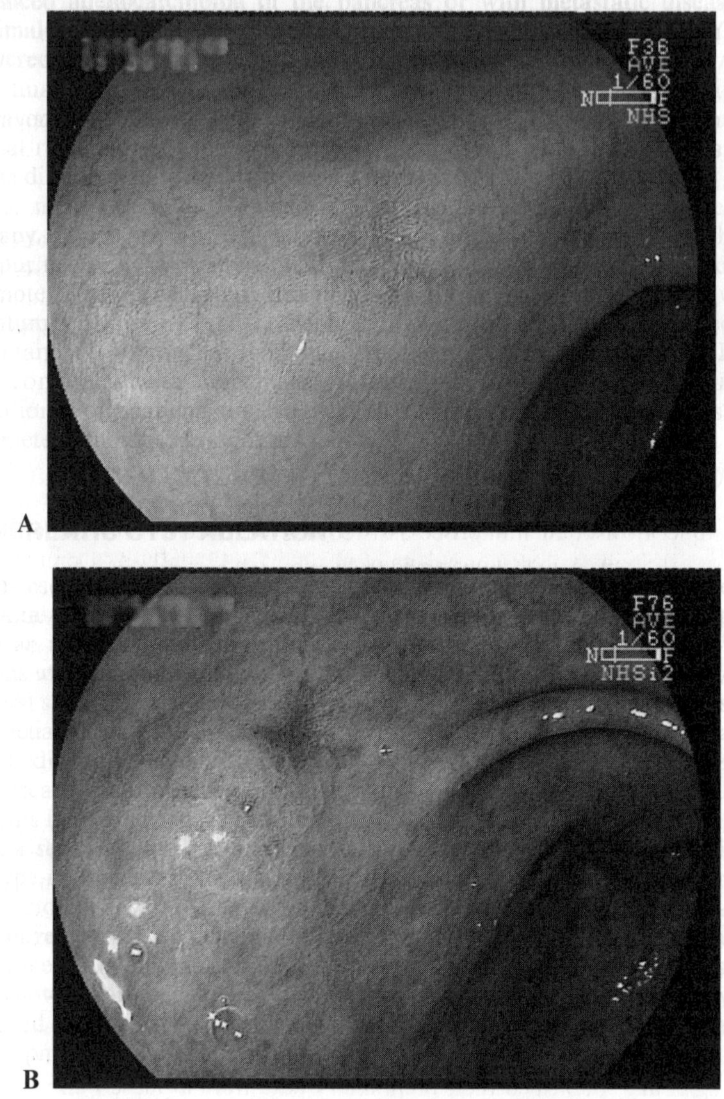

Figure 3 (and opposite)   EGC, type 0-IIc, well-differentiated adenocarcinoma (tub 1), m.A: Conventional endoscopic image; **B**: FICE image, distant view without magnification; **C**: FICE image with magnification, vascular pattern is clearly seen

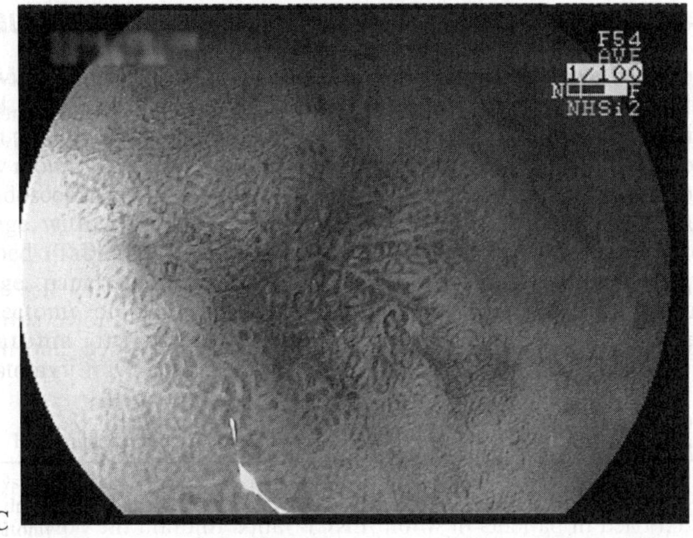

C

interrupted and enlarged are considered submucosal cancer. Ulcerative lesions surrounded by a tumorous bank, or those with folds that are elevated and merged, are considered advanced cancer[17,18].

EUS is useful in combination with conventional endoscopy for staging of the depth of invasion of EGC[18]. It is also useful for evaluating perigastric lymph node metastasis and direct infiltration of adjacent organs[19]. EUS is most useful for determining the depth of invasion when the tumour is histologically differentiated and endoscopically of the small elevated type of EGC[20]. Endosonographic irregular narrowing and a budding sign of more than 1 mm in depth in the third layer (submucosa) are useful for the diagnosis of submucosal invasion in gastric cancers that are diagnosed as mucosal cancers without ulcerous change on endoscopy[21].

Determination of extent of tumour

Even though targeted areas of the mucosa can be removed precisely by ESD (the details of the technique for doing so are described below), complete resection of lesions cannot be expected without determining the extent of EGC. The margin of the tumour should be carefully determined, since the true tumour margin may be wider than that on conventional endoscopic evaluation. Chromoendoscopy, which is often carried out by spraying dyes such as indigo carmine after thoroughly washing out the mucus, is useful for determining the extent of a tumour by clarifying its margins. Observation of fine structure and fine vasculature using a magnifying endoscope combined with NBI or FICE is also particularly useful for determining tumour margins.

ENDOSCOPIC TREATMENT OF EGC

Using the conventional method of endoscopic mucosal resection (EMR), it is often difficult to determine with precision the range of mucosa to be resected. In addition, it is often necessary to perform multiple snaring procedures to remove lesions, due to the limitation in size of mucosa that can be resected at one snaring. There is thus significant risk of piecemeal resection for lesions measuring 10 mm or larger[22,23].

ESD (Figure 4)

ESD is a novel technique that overcomes the limitations of EMR, enabling more reliable and accurate resection of EGC. The technique for incision of the mucosa surrounding the lesion using a needle knife for precise determination of the area to be removed was first reported by Hirao et al.[24]. Procedures common to various techniques of ESD include incision of the mucosa surrounding a lesion and removal of the mucosa by submucosal dissection using electrosurgical knives instead of snaring. With the ESD technique, the mucosa is incised along freely drawn lines of incision, resulting in a high probability of resection of lesions in one piece regardless of their size and location (Figure 5). However, ESD requires more training and skill and takes a longer time to perform than snaring[25–28].

Here is a brief description of the techniques used. Prior to ESD, it is important to observe the margins of a lesion closely and identify the affected area using chromoendoscopy with indigo carmine spray or magnifying endoscopy whenever necessary. As a first step, marks are placed on the surrounding intact mucosa in circumference about 5 mm apart from the margins of the lesion. These marks are usually made with coagulation current using the tip of a knife. Then, the diseased mucosa is, along with the incision line marked beforehand, elevated by submucosal injection. Physiological saline can be used for submucosal injection. However, sodium hyaluronate solution has been proven to maintain submucosal elevation for a longer time, and is therefore useful for providing safety margins for the incision and dissection of the mucosa during ESD[26,27,29–31]. A small amount of epinephrine and indigo carmine are often mixed into the local injection fluid.

The mucosa is incised along the outside of the marks using various endoscopic dissection instruments including a needle knife, while ample mucosal elevation is maintained. After mucosal incision, a knife is inserted through the incised layer of the mucosa and the submucosal tissue is dissected using various dissection instruments to remove the diseased mucosa. Finally, incision along the circumference of the mucosa surrounding the lesion is completed and dissection is performed through the entire submucosa under the diseased part to remove the lesion in one piece. Various types of ESD knives are used in Japan. The principal ESD knives are shown in Figure 6.

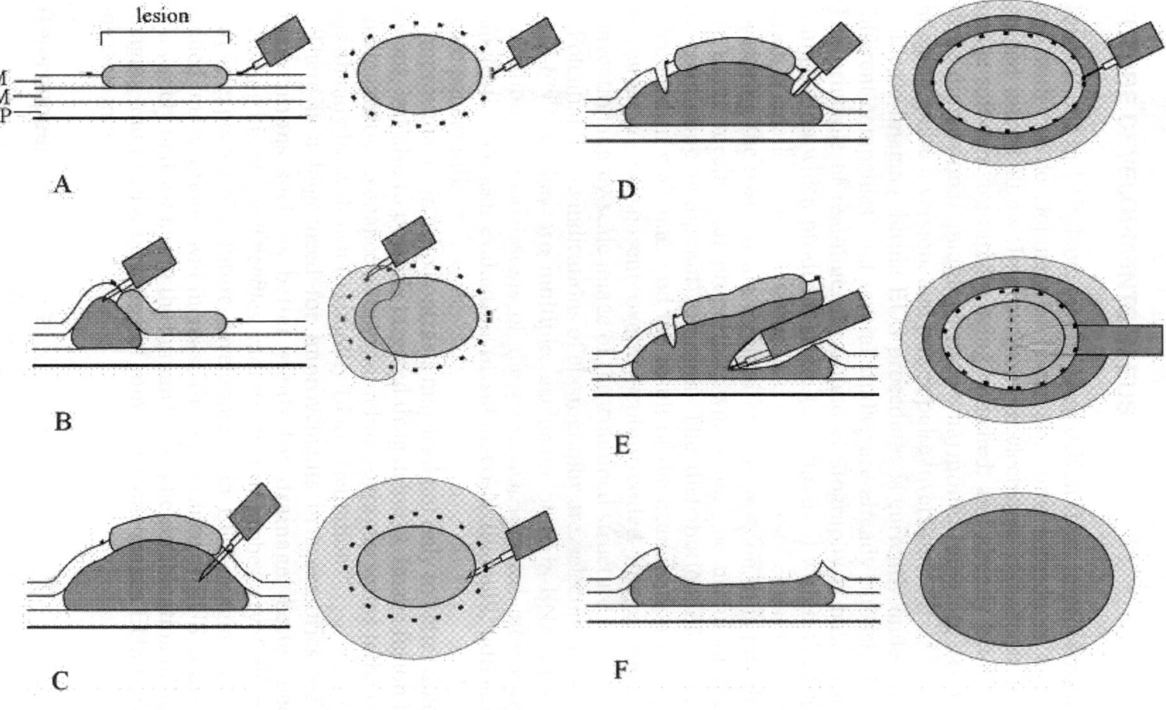

Figure 4 Step-by-step procedures of ESD. **A**: Marking placements around the lesion; **B**: submucosal injection started from the distant edge; **C**: lifting of the entire lesion with submucosal injection; **D**: mucosal incision around the lesion; **E**: submucosal dissection with a knife; **F**: complete en-bloc resection of the lesion

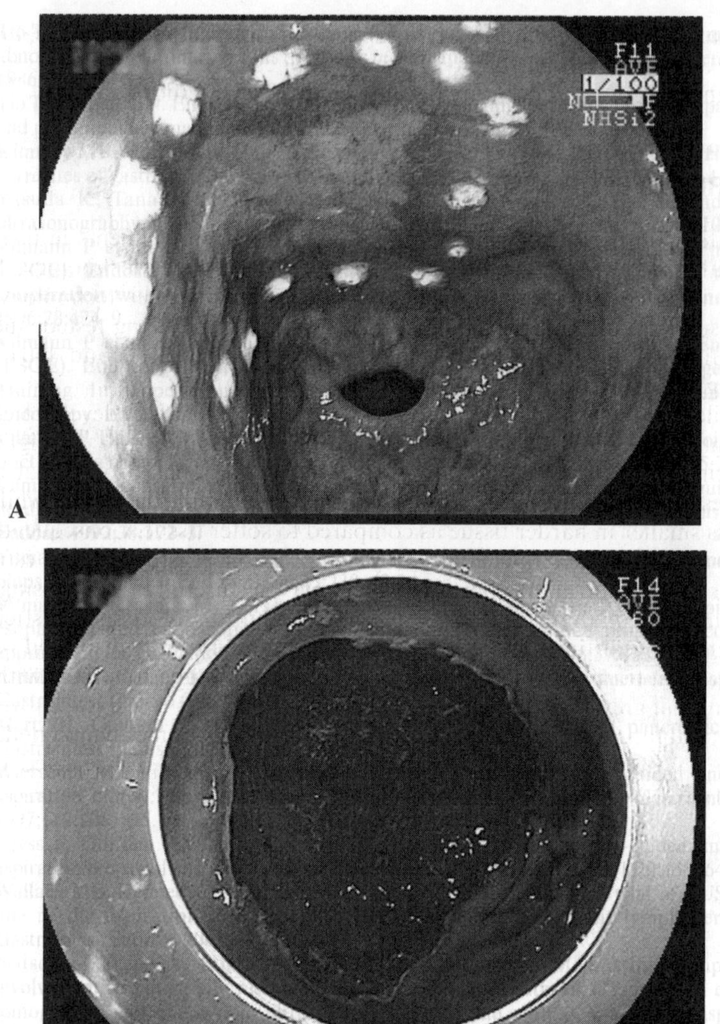

Figure 5 (and opposite) ESD for an EGC (type 0-IIc). **A**: Marking placements under observation using FICE; **B**: mucosal defect after ESD; **C**: resected specimen using ESD

ESD using sodium hyaluronate and a small-calibre-tip transparent (ST) hood (DH-15GR; Fujinon, Saitama, Japan)[27]

This method, developed by the author, utilizes long-lasting submucosal elevation for safe incision and dissection of the mucosa and submucosa using a needle knife. Submucosal injection of sodium hyaluronate is used to maintain

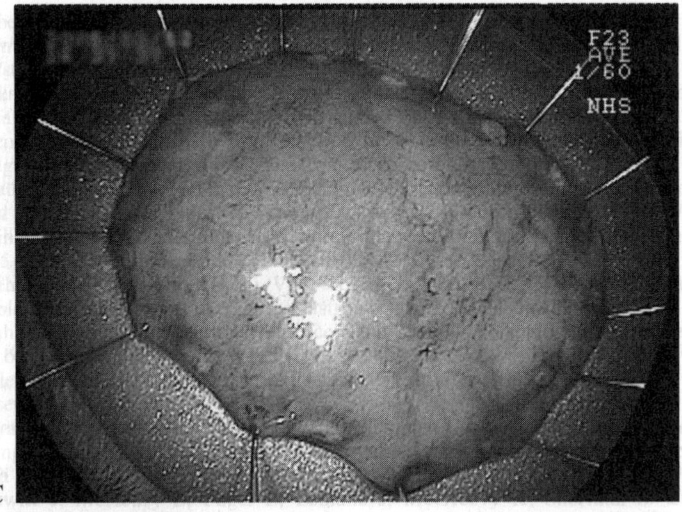

sufficient thickening of the submucosal tissue. An ST hood (Figure 7A) is used to open up the incised mucosa as a substitute for countertraction and also aids control of the knife (Figure 7B). This method enables precise determination of both the lateral and vertical margins to be resected, since all procedures including submucosal incision are carried out under direct visualization.

For successful ESD, control of bleeding during the procedure is very important. A haemostatic forceps is useful for controlling bleeding during ESD. When blood vessels are found during dissection of the submucosal layer, they should be isolated by dissecting the surrounding submucosal tissue. They should then be coagulated using a haemostatic forceps with application of 60–80 W in soft coagulation mode. If bleeding occurs during dissection, bleeding points should be immediately identified by washing the blood with a water jet, and the bleeding vessel should be grasped and coagulated with the coagulation forceps.

A Flush knife is a special needle knife developed by Dr Toyonaga and Fujinon. For this knife, the appropriate length of needle can be selected from among 1, 1.5, 2, 2.5, and 3 mm based on the procedure (Figure 6F). Another unique feature of this knife is the water jet function through the knife sheath. Water or saline can be injected through the Flush knife using a pump for the water jet. A diluted sodium hyaluronate solution can be injected through the knife for submucosal injection during dissection using a 10 ml syringe as well.

HANDLING OF RESECTED SPECIMENS

According to the 2nd English edition of the Japanese Classification of Gastric Carcinoma[8], specimens obtained by endoscopic or laparoscopic mucosal resection should be handled in the following manner: the specimen is spread

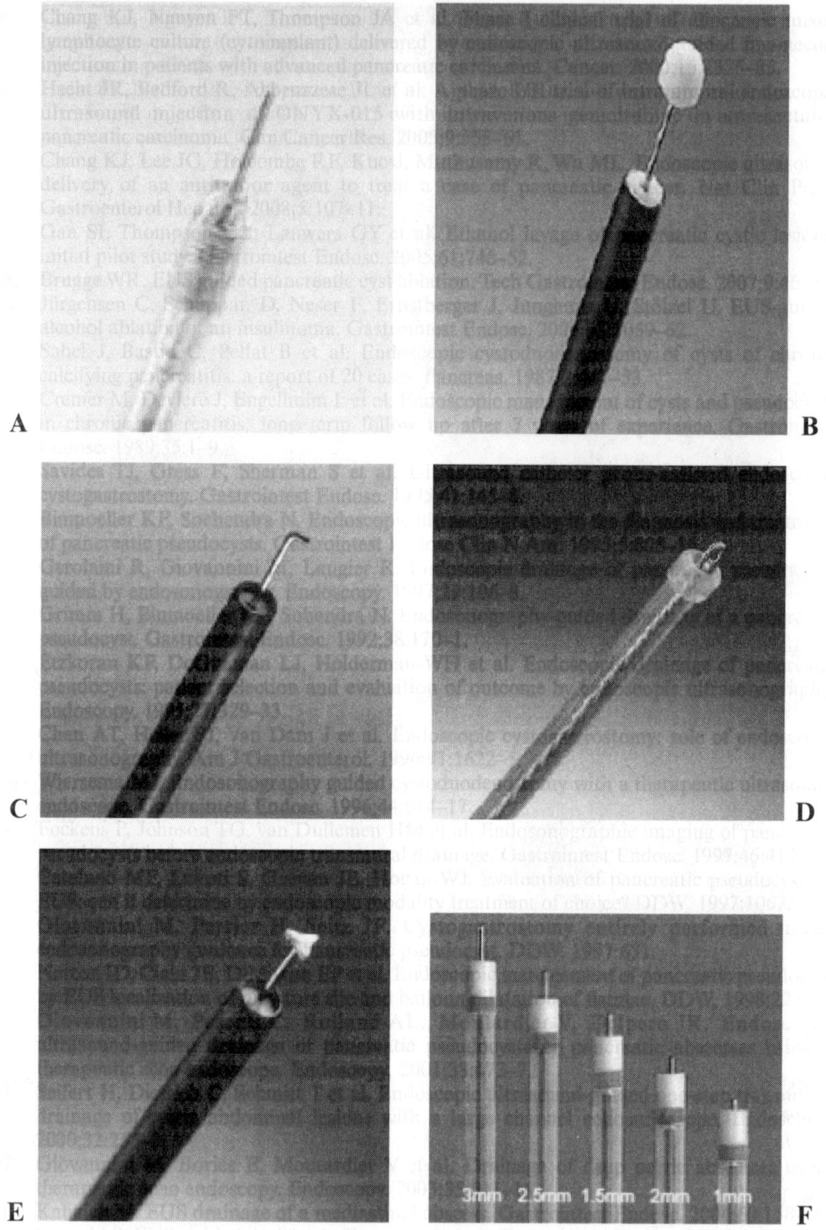

Figure 6 Several kinds of ESD knives. **A**: Needle knife; **B**: IT knife; **C**: Hook knife; **D**: Flex knife; **E**: Triangle-tip knife; **F**: Flush knife

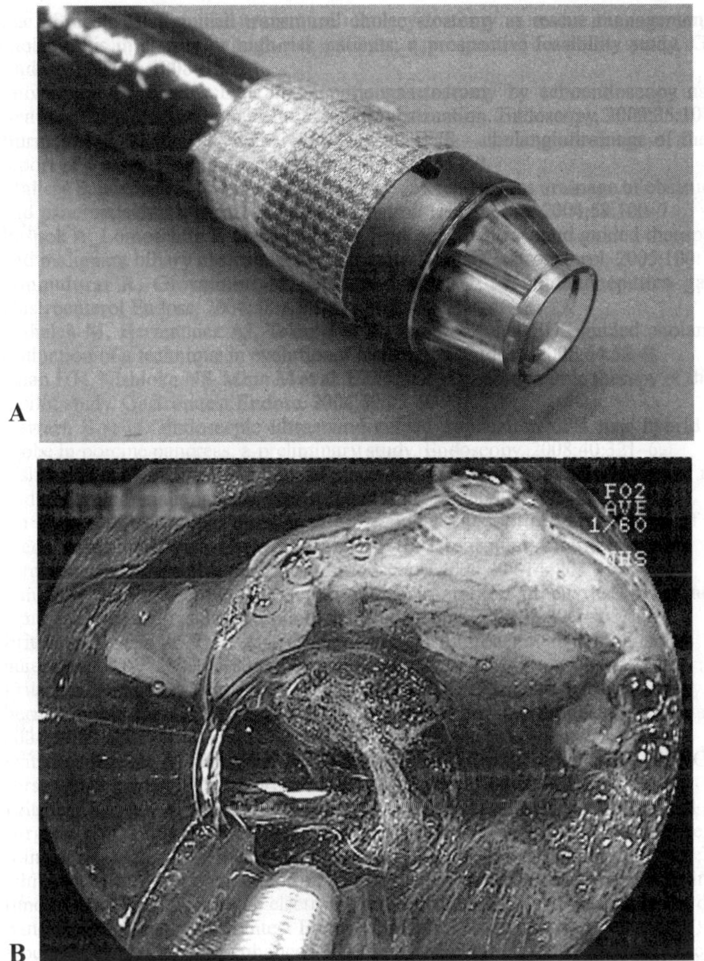

Figure 7 A small-caliber-tip transparent hood (ST hood). **A**: ST hood (DH-15GR, Fujinon) attached to the tip of an endoscope; **B**: incised mucosa is opened up with the tip of the ST hood

out, pinned on flat cork, and fixed in formalin solution. The size of the specimen, the size and shape of the tumour, and the margins should be recorded on a schematic diagram. The proximal cut end is indicated by an arrow, if possible. Fixed materials should be sectioned serially at 2 mm intervals parallel to a line that includes the closest margin of resection of the specimen.

HISTOLOGICAL EXAMINATION

The histological type and largest dimension of the tumour and the presence or absence of ulceration (UL), lymphatic invasion (ly), and venous invasion (v) should be recorded. The depth of invasion (M, SM1, SM2) is determined and recorded only when the vertical margin (VM) is negative (SM1: submucosal invasion <0.5 mm, SM2: invasion $\geqslant 0.5$ mm).

The lateral margin (LM) should be assessed, and if LM is negative, the length (mm) of the free margin or the number of normal tubules in the margin is recorded. Tumour extent, together with depth of invasion, should be recorded on a schematic diagram.

Curative potential of mucosal resection

Resection is considered curative if the following criteria are met: depth M (mucosa), histologically determined papillary adenocarcinoma (pap) or tubular adenocarcinoma (tub), no ulcer or ulcer scar in the tumour, VM (–), no tumour cells within 1 mm of LM, and neither lymphatic nor venous invasion.

CONCLUSIONS

It is recognized that endoscopic treatment of EGC, when performed with the appropriate indications, can yield curability equivalent to that of surgical resection. As regards postoperative quality of life, endoscopic therapy is preferred as long as complete cure is obtained. To perform endoscopic therapy without reducing its curability, preoperative diagnosis, appropriate standards for determining whether this treatment is indicated, appropriate technique, and evaluation of curability based on detailed pathological examination of resected specimens are important.

Innovations such as the high-definition endoscope, magnifying endoscope, NBI, FICE, endocytoscopy, and confocal laser endomicroscopy can enhance early detection and accurate diagnosis of gastric cancer. In addition, innovations in techniques of endoscopic treatment such as ESD have enabled reliable endoscopic treatment for EGC.

References

1. Inoue K, Tobe T, Kan N et al. Problems in the definition and treatment of early gastric cancer. Br J Surg. 1991;78:818–21.
2. Onodera H, Tokunaga A, Yoshiyuki T et al. Surgical outcome of 483 patients with early gastric cancer: prognosis, postoperative morbidity and mortality, and gastric remnant cancer. Hepatogastroenterology. 2004;51:82–5.
3. Yamamoto H. Technology insight: endoscopic submucosal dissection of gastrointestinal neoplasms. Nat Clin Pract Gastroenterol Hepatol. 2007;4:511–20.
4. Seto Y, Nagawa H, Muto T. Impact of lymph node metastasis on survival with early gastric cancer. World J Surg. 1997;21:186–89; discussion 190.
5. Adachi Y, Shiraishi N, Kitano S. Modern treatment of early gastric cancer: review of the Japanese experience. Dig Surg. 2002;19:333–9.
6. Kunisaki C, Shimada H, Takahashi M et al. Prognostic factors in early gastric cancer. Hepatogastroenterology. 2001;48:294–8.

7. Gotoda T, Yanagisawa A, Sasako M et al. Incidence of lymph node metastasis from early gastric cancer: estimation with a large number of cases at two large centers. Gastric Cancer. 2000;3:219–225.

8. Japanese Gastric Cancer. Japanese Classification of Gastric Carcinoma, 2nd English edn. Gastric Cancer. 1998;1:10–24.

9. Yamamoto H, Kita H. Endoscopic therapy of early gastric cancer. Best Pract Res Clin Gastroenterol. 2005;19:909–26.

10. Triantafillidis JK, Cheracakis P. Diagnostic evaluation of patients with early gastric cancer – a literature review. Hepatogastroenterology. 2004;51:618–24.

11. Machida H, Sano Y, Hamamoto Y et al. Narrow-band imaging in the diagnosis of colorectal mucosal lesions: a pilot study. Endoscopy. 2004;36:1094–8.

12. Yao K, Matsui T, Iwashita A. [Clinical application of magnification endoscopy with NBI for diagnosis of early gastric cancer]. Nippon Shokakibyo Gakkai Zasshi. 2007;104:782–9.

13. Adler A, Pohl H, Papanikolaou IS et al. A prospective randomised study on narrow-band imaging versus conventional colonoscopy for adenoma detection: does narrow-band imaging induce a learning effect? Gut. 2008;57:59–64.

14. Kaltenbach T, Friedland S, Soetikno R. A randomised tandem colonoscopy trial of narrow band imaging versus white light examination to compare neoplasia miss rates. Gut. 2008;57:1406–12.

15. Rex DK, Helbig CC. High yields of small and flat adenomas with high-definition colonoscopes using either white light or narrow band imaging. Gastroenterology. 2007;133:42–7.

16. Osawa H, Yoshizawa M, Yamamoto H et al. Optimal band imaging system can facilitate detection of changes in depressed-type early gastric cancer. Gastrointest Endosc. 2008;67:226–34.

17. Sano T, Okuyama Y, Kobori O et al. Early gastric cancer. Endoscopic diagnosis of depth of invasion. Dig Dis Sci. 1990;35:1340–4.

18. Yanai H, Matsumoto Y, Harada T et al. Endoscopic ultrasonography and endoscopy for staging depth of invasion in early gastric cancer: a pilot study. Gastrointest Endosc. 1997;46:212–16.

19. Akahoshi K, Misawa T, Fujishima H et al. Preoperative evaluation of gastric cancer by endoscopic ultrasound. Gut. 1991;32:479–82.

20. Akahoshi K, Chijiwa Y, Hamada S et al. Pretreatment staging of endoscopically early gastric cancer with a 15 MHz ultrasound catheter probe. Gastrointest Endosc. 1998;48:470–6.

21. Matsumoto Y, Yanai H, Tokiyama H et al. Endoscopic ultrasonography for diagnosis of submucosal invasion in early gastric cancer. J Gastroenterol. 2000;35:326–31.

22. Inoue H, Takeshita K, Hori H et al. Endoscopic mucosal resection with a cap-fitted panendoscope for esophagus, stomach, and colon mucosal lesions. Gastrointest Endosc. 1993;39:58–62.

23. Tada M, Murakami A, Karita M et al. Endoscopic resection of early gastric cancer. Endoscopy. 1993;25:445–50.

24. Hirao M, Masuda K, Asanuma T et al. Endoscopic resection of early gastric cancer and other tumors with local injection of hypertonic saline-epinephrine. Gastrointest Endosc. 1988;34:264–9.

25. Soetikno RM, Gotoda T, Nakanishi Y et al. Endoscopic mucosal resection. Gastrointest Endosc. 2003;57:567–79.

26. Yamamoto H, Kawata H, Sunada K et al. Success rate of curative endoscopic mucosal resection with circumferential mucosal incision assisted by submucosal injection of sodium hyaluronate. Gastrointest Endosc. 2002;56:507–12.

27. Yamamoto H, Kawata H, Sunada K et al. Successful en-bloc resection of large superficial tumors in the stomach and colon using sodium hyaluronate and small-caliber-tip transparent hood. Endoscopy. 2003;35:690–4.

28. Ohkuwa M, Hosokawa K, Boku N et al. New endoscopic treatment for intramucosal gastric tumors using an insulated-tip diathermic knife. Endoscopy. 2001;33:221–6.

29. Yamamoto H, Yube T, Isoda N et al. A novel method of endoscopic mucosal resection using sodium hyaluronate. Gastrointest Endosc. 1999;50:251–6.

30. Fujishiro M, Yahagi N, Kashimura K et al. Different mixtures of sodium hyaluronate and their ability to create submucosal fluid cushions for endoscopic mucosal resection. Endoscopy. 2004;36:584–9.
31. Fujishiro M, Yahagi N, Kashimura K et al. Comparison of various submucosal injection solutions for maintaining mucosal elevation during endoscopic mucosal resection. Endoscopy. 2004;36:579–83.

Section III
Small bowel and bile ducts

Chair: G GAY and Z DÖBRÖNTE

- All detected polyps should be removed; however, age of the patient and co-morbidities in order to avoid over-treatment should also be considered.
- Not all polyps must be removed endoscopically, there is a small fraction of polyps that are better managed surgically, and over-ambitious endoscopists should not insist on removing all of them.
- Endoscopists should know their abilities and limitations; they should know their endoscopic equipment, especially electrosurgical.
- Histologists should be provided with high-quality material, not destroyed, not cut into pieces.
- Completeness of removal should be assessed both endoscopically and histologically.
- Polypectomy should be performed in one piece whenever possible.
- The six o'clock rule should be remembered (positioning of the polyp in the endoscopic view for removal).
- When cold snare polypectomy is performed, there is no need to inflate the lesion, and lifting should not be done.
- When hot-snare polypectomy is done, coagulation current should be used whenever possible.
- Bowel should always be de-sulfated before polypectomy.
- Passing the tissue for polypectomy should be optimally done by the endoscopist and not by accompanying nurse.

The recommendation decision rule concerning method of polyps removal is presented in Figure 2. Different scenarios are immediately modified to fit settings depending on the experience, availability of education and other factors.

Further diagnostic procedure depends on the histopathology report, which should contain: histopathological type of the polyp, dysplasia grade in case of adenomas, and completeness of removal. The histopathological algorithm is presented in Figure 2.

Malignant foci within adenomas require more specific information, including distance of cancer focus from the resection line, presence of lymphatic and blood vessels as well as cancer differentiation grade. If malignant foci are present within adenomas, endoscopic removal can be regarded as sufficient only if removal was not piecemeal and invasion was not deeper than submucosa. Detailed information on this issue can be found elsewhere. In patients in whom polyps have been removed, used surveillance in the family recommendations concerning this step are changing recently in the direction of less intensive surveillance, as compared to previous years. Recent recommendations are presented in Table 1. These recommendations are valid only if high-quality colonoscopy has been performed, the entire clean colon without polyps has been obtained, and only if cleaning was credited.

4
Small bowel: standards and innovations: capsule endoscopy, push enteroscopy and push-and-pull enteroscopy in single- and double-balloon technique

A. MAY

INTRODUCTION

Until only a few years ago it was not possible to access most of the small bowel using endoscopic techniques that avoided the need for surgery. Video capsule endoscopy and balloon enteroscopy thus represent decisive breakthroughs in this field. Capsule endoscopy is a safe method, which in most cases allows endoscopic visualization of the entire small bowel. A substantial disadvantage of the method is the inability to obtain histological samples and carry out endoscopic treatments. In addition, the interpretation of non-specific findings is not easy in some cases, and requires confirmation and checking using a second procedure.

Flexible enteroscopy using push enteroscopy and balloon enteroscopy is a more invasive procedure in comparison with capsule endoscopy. However, it provides all the advantages of conventional endoscopy. Push enteroscopy became established in the 1980s, but is associated with only a limited depth of penetration into the small bowel. This limitation was overcome through the development of balloon enteroscopy[1]. In optimal cases the entire small bowel, or at least considerable proportions of it, can be visualized using balloon enteroscopy (usually by combining oral and anal examinations). Depending on the endoscopist's level of experience, the rate of complete enteroscopy using the double-balloon method is around 80% (maximum 86%)[2,3]. With single-balloon enteroscopy the rates are currently up to a maximum of 25%[4]. In 2001 the double-balloon enteroscopy (DBE) system developed by Dr Yamamoto was presented for the first time in Japan, and in 2003 by our own research group in Germany[5,6]. In the meantime the system has become established throughout the world for diagnostic and therapeutic small-bowel examinations, and in Germany in particular it is now being used universally in clinical routine work throughout the country. In addition to the classic indication for small-bowel endoscopy, the DBE technique also has a variety of other potential uses – e.g. in difficult colonoscopies, or for access to the pancreatic and biliary tract in patients with a surgically modified gastrointestinal tract, and for access to the stomach in patients who have undergone obesity surgery. Another balloon enteroscopy system was recently introduced that is equipped with only one balloon at the tip of the overtube and is therefore known as single-balloon enteroscopy (SBE)[4]. The two systems and their potential clinical applications are briefly presented below. The discussion on balloon enteroscopy – double- versus single-balloon technique – is of main interest, therefore this chapter is focused on this new topic.

CAPSULE ENDOSCOPY

Details of capsule data and the performance of capsule endoscopy examinations have been published elsewhere previously[7]. On the basis of the published data, identifying mid-gastrointestinal bleeding as the cause of obscure bleeding appears to be the most suitable indication for the procedure. Published reports have described success rates in the range of 48–76% with capsule endoscopy in patients with mid-gastrointestinal bleeding. Other potential indications include suspected Crohn's disease and polyposis syndromes such as familial adenomatosis or Peutz–Jeghers syndrome. Treatment-refractory coeliac disease is also a conceivable indication[8].

PUSH ENTEROSCOPY (PE)

Push video enteroscopes are 230–250 cm long devices (dependent on type and manufacturer) and might be used with a stiff overtube (100–120 cm) to prevent looping of the enteroscope in the stomach. While initial studies showed an increase in depth of insertion with the use of an overtube[8,9], later studies with graded stiffness enteroscopes have questioned the additional value of the overtube[10,11]; therefore many units no longer use it in routine practice. PE for the lower digestive tract is not commonly performed, because insertion depth of colonoscopy with ileoscopy appears equivalent to lower PE[6].

DOUBLE-BALLOON ENTEROSCOPY (DBE)

The double-balloon enteroscopy system (Fujinon, Inc., Saitama, Japan) consists of a high-resolution video endoscope with a working length of 200 cm and a flexible overtube made of polyurethane. Latex balloons are attached at the tip of the enteroscopy and also on the overtube, and can be filled with air or emptied using a pressure-controlled pump. The principle of the DBE technique is based on alternating pushing and pulling manoeuvres, allowing the small bowel to be threaded onto the overtube step by step[4,5]. Two different types of device are currently available with the double-balloon system: the EN450-P5 model, with a working channel of 2.2 mm and an outer diameter of 8.5 mm; and the EN450-T5 model, with a working channel of 2.8 mm and an outer diameter of 9.4 mm. The corresponding overtubes have diameters of 12.2 and 13.2 mm, respectively, with an overall length of 145 cm.

SINGLE-BALLOON ENTEROSCOPY (SBE)

The single-balloon enteroscopy system was introduced only recently (Olympus, Inc., Tokyo, Japan). The enteroscope (XSIF Q260Y) is also a high-resolution video endoscope, with a working length of 200 cm. The enteroscope is equipped with a working channel 2.8 mm in diameter, and its outer diameter is 9.2 mm. The overtube has an overall length of 140 cm, consists of silicone, and has a latex-free balloon made of silicone at its distal end. In contrast to the DBE system, a balloon is not attached to the tip of the enteroscope, and stable positioning in the small bowel is achieved during withdrawal of the scope by angling the tip of the endoscope. Insufflation of the overtube balloon is carried out using a pressure-controlled pump.

In principle the DBE system can of course also be used as a SBE system, by dispensing with the balloon attached to the enteroscope tip[13,14].

EXAMINATION PROCEDURE

For both DBE and SBE the patient only needs to fast before the oral examination (approximately 12 h for food, approximately 4 h for clear liquids). For the anal examination, laxative measures are necessary in the same way as in colonoscopy. Laxative measures before oral examinations may be useful in patients with suspected stenoses or diabetic neuropathy with delayed transit.

The examination itself is carried out either with conventional sedoanalgesia or with propofol sedation. General anaesthesia with intubation is not customary in Germany and is restricted to individual cases – e.g. in children.

Depending on experience, radiological fluoroscopy can be used as an aid in balloon enteroscopy. Particularly when adhesions are expected following prior abdominal surgery, fluoroscopy can be very useful. When stenoses are expected – e.g. in patients with Crohn's disease – radiology is certainly useful, as the radiographic contrast image allows good assessment of the complexity of impassable stenoses. When endoscopic retrograde cholangiopancreatography (ERCP) is being carried out with balloon enteroscopy, radiographic imaging is of course necessary in any case[2].

Following positive reports on the use of CO_2 insufflation in colonoscopy and ERCP, a prospective two-centre study has now been published that has demonstrated substantial advantages of CO_2 insufflation also for DBE[15]. Patient comfort is markedly improved, as reflected in reduced perception of pain. In addition, the depth of penetration appears to be markedly improved. Despite these positive data, the use of CO_2 has not yet become generally established, however. This could change if experience is confirmed by further studies.

INDICATION FOR BALLOON ENDOSCOPY

On the basis of the extensive published data on DBE and on the European Guidelines for small bowel endoscopy, suspected or known mid-gastrointestinal bleeding represents the principal indication for the procedure[16–22]. The same certainly also applies to SBE[4,23], as there is no difference in the indications for the two enteroscopy methods. Lesions that have been discovered using other imaging procedures, such as magnetic resonance enteroclysis (MR Sellink), can be diagnostically checked using balloon enteroscopy and histologically confirmed if necessary. If there is a suspicion of small-bowel obstruction, balloon endoscopy is preferable to capsule endoscopy as a diagnostic step, in view of the risk of capsule retention[24].

In addition to haemostatic procedures, balloon endoscopy can also be used in the deep small bowel to carry out resection of superficial or polypoid lesions, as well as for balloon dilation of stenoses, preoperative marking of pathological findings, foreign-body removal (e.g. retained capsules, parts of dentures, plastic prostheses, etc.) and also in a few cases for implantation of self-expanding metal stents[3,16,17,21,25,26].

As mentioned above, DBE is also suitable for obtaining access to a surgically modified gastrointestinal tract – for example, in ERCP after Billroth II operations or gastric resection with Roux-en-Y reconstruction[27,28], as well as for access to the biliary system or residual stomach after obesity surgery[29]. Another area of application appears to be difficult ileocolonoscopy[30–32]. For colonoscopy and ERCP there have also been positive reports of experience in the form of case series and a case report using the single-balloon technique[13,14].

Mid-gastrointestinal bleeding

Mid-gastrointestinal bleeding is defined as small-bowel bleeding located between the papilla and the ileocaecal valve[33]. The first comparative studies of capsule endoscopy and DBE showed that the two methods had a similar diagnostic yield[34–36]. In comparison with push enteroscopy, a much higher diagnostic yield can be achieved with DBE, as expected, since much more of the small bowel can be visualized[1,37]. No studies comparing DBE with SBE have so far been published. The high diagnostic yield of DBE, at around 60–80%, is also associated with a high percentage of direct therapeutic implications for the patient[3,16–18,20]. Most publications on DBE have reported a high rate of endoscopic interventions, at between 35% and 65%. The first original studies in Asia on SBE show a slightly lower diagnostic yield of around 40–50%[4,23], while the rate of endoscopic interventions was only 5–20%. However, the data are still too limited in comparison with DBE for a valid assessment to be possible. In addition, it is well known that angiodysplasias, which can generally be well treated endoscopically, are much more frequent in the western hemisphere than in Asia. Only preliminary data are so far available concerning the effectiveness of endoscopic therapy, e.g. after haemostasis, in relation to the long-term course for patients in stabilizing haemoglobin values and reducing the need for blood transfusions. However, positive experience has been reported with push enteroscopy with regard to the endoscopic treatment of patients with mid-gastrointestinal bleeding[38,39], and it can be assumed that the same will also apply in balloon enteroscopy. However, studies with longer follow-up periods and larger numbers of patients would be desirable.

The algorithms generally proposed for the diagnostic work-up in mid-gastrointestinal bleeding therefore depend on the level of the users' experience and the technical facilities available. There is general agreement that, after a negative oesophagogastroduodenoscopy (OGD) and colonoscopy, capsule endoscopy should be the third examination used in the diagnostic work-up of patients with mid-gastrointestinal bleeding. Depending on the capsule results, it can be decided whether balloon enteroscopy is needed and which access route (oral or anal) should be used, and any treatment steps required can be planned[2]. Before elaborate small-bowel diagnosis, however, OGD and gastroscopy should be repeated, as it has been shown that simply repeating these two examinations can identify a bleeding source in up to 20% of cases[7]. When capsule endoscopy is negative, and there is confirmed overt or occult gastrointestinal bleeding, balloon enteroscopy should be attempted as the next step. If the case primarily involves active bleeding, with a high probability that a therapeutic intervention will be needed, enteroscopy should precede capsule endoscopy. The same also applies to patients with a surgically modified gastrointestinal tract, since the afferent loop after a Roux-en-Y reconstruction is not usually visualized with the capsule, for example. In addition, in patients with signs of intestinal obstruction or with stenoses suspected on the basis of clinical signs or other imaging procedures, balloon enteroscopy takes priority due to the risk of capsule retention[2].

Crohn's disease

Balloon enteroscopy is certainly not one of the standard procedures in the initial diagnosis of Crohn's disease or for follow-up examinations in patients with known Crohn's disease. Balloon enteroscopy has a place only in patients with obstructive Crohn's disease, as it allows dilation to be carried out. In rare cases, direct visual observation and histological sampling may be required in order to confirm Crohn's carcinoma. In addition, the inflammatory components in a stenotically altered segment of the small bowel can be more reliably assessed with direct visualization, and this is important for the patient's subsequent drug treatment. The need for endoscopic dilation treatment or surgical treatment can also be effectively assessed[2].

Polyposis syndrome

Patients with polyposis syndromes – familial adenomatous polyposis (FAP), Peutz–Jeghers syndrome – in the colon and/or small bowel usually undergo surgery, and therefore often have considerable numbers of adhesions. Balloon enteroscopy is therefore difficult in these patients, and complete enteroscopy will not always be possible. Balloon enteroscopy therefore has a place here for therapeutic endoscopy with polypectomy. In FAP patients with evidence of duodenal adenomas, screening should be carried out with capsule endoscopy, as the adenomas mainly grow very superficially and are best detected with this method. Peutz–Jeghers polyps usually consist of polypoid lesions that can be diagnosed both with capsule endoscopy and also with radiographic imaging – e.g. MR Sellink. As small-bowel involvement can be expected in more than 90% of patients with Peutz–Jeghers syndrome, balloon enteroscopy can be used as the first diagnostic procedure, with an expectation that treatment will be needed, in symptomatic Peutz–Jeghers patients (those with anaemia and/or obstruction)[40].

Small-bowel tumours

The frequency of small-bowel tumours in patients with mid-gastrointestinal bleeding is between 5% and 10%. Up to 60% of the tumours are malignant[41]. Balloon enteroscopy represents the treatment of choice in patients with suspected small-bowel tumour, due to the facility for histological sampling. In treatment-refractory coeliac disease, balloon enteroscopy is similarly the treatment of choice, due to the availability of histological sampling for identifying T-cell lymphomas[42]. The same also applies to the staging of gastrointestinal lymphomas beyond the stomach – although there are as yet insufficient data for balloon enteroscopy to be used as the standard examination.

COMPLICATIONS

On the basis of the published data, including the German double-balloon registry (including just under 4000 DBE procedures), relevant complications in diagnostic DBE can be expected in approximately 1% of cases. The most severe complication here is certainly pancreatitis, with a risk of approximately 0.3% in oral DBE. As in conventional endoscopy, the risk is higher in therapeutic enteroscopy, at around 3–4%[43,44]. In findings similar to those of the prospective Munich colon polypectomy study, it has been found that the complication risk (bleeding and perforation) may reach as much as 10%, particularly with large, broad-based polyps[25]. Experience is indispensable here in order to minimize complications.

With regard to the mortality rate associated with DBE, the only data available are from the German double-balloon registry. The mortality rate here is 0.05% (death after pancreatitis and complicated postoperative course after perforation during polypectomy for a small-bowel polyp).

Insufficient data are currently available with regard to the expected complication rates in diagnostic and therapeutic SBE. Perforation as a severe complication of a diagnostic examination has been reported in only one of the two original studies that have been published to date (one of 37 examinations in 27 patients)[23]. In the other study[4], a deep mucosal tear was described, which was treated with clips (one of 78 examinations in 41 patients). This was caused by the flexed endoscope tip during advancement of the overtube. It is conceivable that this inverted endoscope tip technique might lead to a higher rate of relevant mucosal injuries, but due to the limited numbers of cases the question cannot as yet be answered.

CONTRAINDICATIONS FOR BALLOON ENDOSCOPY

The contraindications for balloon endoscopy correspond to those for conventional endoscopy in the upper and lower gastrointestinal tract. Adhesions are not contraindications for the examination, but represent limitations of it, as the depth of penetration into the small bowel can be restricted by fixed small-bowel loops. In addition, adhesions can lead to considerable discomfort for the patients during and after the examination. In patients with a latex allergy, 'anti-allergic prophylaxis', comparable with the prophylaxis administered in patients with contrast allergies in ERCP, is advisable when the double-balloon system is used. There are no evidence-based data on the necessity for this measure, however.

SUMMARY

Capsule endoscopy is a safe method, but only a diagnostic tool and therefore excellent for screening. Push enteroscopy is a more invasive procedure than the capsule, but offers all options of conventinal endoscopy including biopsy sampling and endoscopic therapy. The disadvantage of push entroscopy is the limited insertion depth, so that only lesions in the proximal jejunum can be diagnosed and treated endoscopically. Therefore, balloon enteroscopy has become established throughout the world for diagnostic and therapeutic examinations of the small bowel, and is now used universally in clinical routine work in Germany in particular. The main advantages of the method in comparison with other imaging procedures (e.g. capsule endoscopy and MR Sellink) are that it allows histological sampling and endoscopic therapy. With good patient selection, relevant pathological findings can be detected in a high percentage of cases (70–80%) with DBE, leading in turn to direct therapeutic implications for the patient. Endoscopic therapy can be carried out in more than 50% of patients with mid-gastrointestinal bleeding. The complication rates with both diagnostic and therapeutic DBE are acceptably low. The recently introduced technique of SBE represents a simplification of the method, and the initial preliminary data for it have been positive, although the rate of complete enteroscopies appears to be markedly lower. It remains to be seen whether a significant reduction in the detection rate for relevant findings is associated with the method. On the basis of the currently available data, DBE must continue to be regarded as the gold standard procedure at present. Larger prospective studies on SBE, and above all prospective studies comparing the two systems, are awaited before conclusive assessments can be made.

References

1. May A, Nachbar L, Schneider M, Ell C. Prospective comparison of push enteroscopy and push-and-pull enteroscopy in patients with suspected small-bowel bleeding. Am J Gastroenterol. 2006;101:2016–24.

2. Pohl J, Blancas JM, Cave D et al. Consensus report of the 2nd International Conference on double balloon endoscopy. Endoscopy. 2008;40:156–60.

3. Yamamoto H, Kita H, Sunada K et al. Clinical outcomes of double-balloon endoscopy for the diagnosis and treatment of small-intestinal diseases. Clin Gastroenterol Hepatol. 2004;2:1010–16.

4. Tsujikawa T, Saitoh Y, Andoh A et al. Novel single-balloon enteroscopy for diagnosis and treatment of the small intestine: preliminary experiences. Endoscopy. 2008;40:11–15.

5. Yamamoto H, Sekine Y, Sato Y et al. Total enteroscopy with a nonsurgical steerable double-balloon method. Gastrointest Endosc. 2001;53:216–20.

6. May A, Nachbar L, Wardak A, Yamamoto H, Ell C. Double-balloon enteroscopy: preliminary experience in patients with obscure gastrointestinal bleeding or chronic abdominal pain. Endoscopy. 2003;35:985–91.

7. Ell C, Remke S, May A et al. The first prospective controlled trial comparing wireless capsule endoscopy with push enteroscopy in chronic gastrointestinal bleeding. Endoscopy. 2002;34:685–9.

8. Mergener K, Ponchon T, Gralnek I et al. Literature review and recommendations for clinical application of small-bowel capsule endoscopy, based on a panel discussion by international experts. Consensus statements for small-bowel capsule endoscopy, 2006/2007. Endoscopy. 2007;39:895–909.

9. Taylor AC, Chen RY, Desmond PV. Use of an overtube for enteroscopy – does it increase depth of insertion? A prospective study of enteroscopy with and without an overtube. Endoscopy. 2001;33:227–30.

10. Iida M, Yamamoto T, Yao T et al. Jejunal endoscopy using a long duodenofiberscope. Gastrointest Endosc. 1986;32:233–6.

11. Keizman D, Brill S, Umansky M et al. Diagnostic yield of routine push enteroscopy with a graded-stiffness enteroscope without overtube. Gastrointest Endosc. 2003;57:877–81.

12. Lin S, Branch MS, Shetzline M. The importance of indication in the diagnostic value of push enteroscopy. Endoscopy. 2003;35:315–21.

13. May A, Nachbar L, Ell C. Push-and-pull enteroscopy using a single-balloon technique for difficult colonoscopy. Endoscopy. 2006;38:395–8.

14. Mönkemüller K, Fry LC, Bellutti M, Neumann H, Malfertheiner P. ERCP using single-balloon instead of double-balloon enteroscopy in patients with Roux-en-Y anastomosis. Endoscopy. 2008;40(Suppl.2):E19–20.

15. Domagk D, Bretthauer M, Lenz P et al. Carbon dioxide insufflation improves intubation depth in double-balloon enteroscopy: a randomized, controlled, double-blind trial. Endoscopy. 2007;39:1064–7.

16. Ell C, May A, Nachbar L et al. Push-and-pull enteroscopy in the small bowel using the double-balloon technique: results of a prospective European multicenter study. Endoscopy. 2005;37:613–16.

17. May A, Nachbar L, Ell C. Double-balloon enteroscopy (push-and-pull enteroscopy) of the small bowel: feasibility and diagnostic and therapeutic yield in patients with suspected small bowel disease. Gastrointest Endosc. 2005;62:62–70.

18. Heine GD, Hadithi M, Groenen MJ, Kuipers EJ, Jacobs MA, Mulder CJ. Double balloon enteroscopy: indications, diagnostic yield, and complications in a series of 275 patients with suspected small-bowel diseases. Endoscopy. 2006;38:42–8.

19. Mehdizadeh S, Ross A, Gerson L et al. What is the learning curve associated with double-balloon enteroscopy? Technical details and early experience in 6 U.S. tertiary care centers. Gastrointest Endosc. 2006;64:740–50.

20. Sun B, Rajan E, Cheng S et al. Diagnostic yield and therapeutic impact of double-balloon enteroscopy in a large cohort of patients with obscure gastrointestinal bleeding. Am J Gastroenterol. 2006;101:2011–15.

21. Zhong J, Ma T, Zhang C et al. A retrospective study of the application on double-balloon enteroscopy in 378 patients with suspected small-bowel diseases. Endoscopy. 2007;39:208–15.
22. Pohl J, Delvaux M, Ell C et al. ESGE Clinical Guidelines Committee European Society of Gastrointestinal Endoscopy (ESGE). Guidelines: flexible enteroscopy for diagnosis and treatment of small-bowel diseases. Endoscopy. 2008;40:609–18.
23. Kawamura T, Yasuda K Tanaka K et al. Clinical evaluation of a newly developed single-balloon enteroscope. Gastrointest Endosc. 2008;68:1112–16.
24. Sunada K, Yamamoto H, Kita H et al. Clinical outcomes of enteroscopy using the double-balloon method for strictures of the small intestine. World J Gastroenterol. 2005;11:1087–9.
25. May A, Nachbar L, Pohl J, Ell C. Endoscopic interventions in the small bowel using double balloon enteroscopy: feasibility and limitations. Am J Gastroenterol. 2007;102:527–35.
26. Lee BI, Choi H, Choi KY et al. Retrieval of a retained capsule endoscope by double-balloon enteroscopy. Gastrointest Endosc. 2005;62:463–5.
27. Haruta H, Yamamoto H, Mizuta K et al. A case of successful enteroscopic balloon dilation for late anastomotic stricture of choledochojejunostomy after living donor liver transplantation. Liver Transplant. 2005;11:1608–10.
28. Aabakken L, Bretthauer M, Line PD. Double-balloon enteroscopy for endoscopic retrograde cholangiography in patients with a Roux-en-Y anastomosis. Endoscopy. 2007;39:1068–71.
29. Kuga R, Safatle-Ribeiro AV, Faintuch J et al. Endoscopic findings in the excluded stomach after Roux-en Y gastric bypass surgery. Arch Surg. 2007;142:942–6.
30. Kaltenbach T, Soetikno R, Friedland S. Use of a double balloon enteroscope facilitates caecal intubation after incomplete colonoscopy with a standard colonoscope. Dig Liver Dis. 2006;38:921–5.
31. Mönkemüller K, Knippig C, Rickes S, Fry LC, Schulze A, Malfertheiner P. Usefulness of the double-balloon enteroscope in colonoscopies performed in patients with previously failed colonoscopy. Scand J Gastroenterol. 2007;42:277–8.
32. Pasha SF, Harrison ME, Das A, Corrado CM, Arnell KN, Leighton JA. Utility of double-balloon colonoscopy for completion of colon examination after incomplete colonoscopy with conventional colonoscope. Gastrointest Endosc. 2007;65:848–53.
33. Ell C, May A. Mid-gastrointestinal bleeding: capsule endoscopy and push-and-pull enteroscopy give rise to a new medical term. Endoscopy. 2006;38:73–5.
34. Hadithi M, Heine GD, Jacobs MA, van Bodegraven AA, Mulder CJ. A prospective study comparing video capsule endoscopy with double-balloon enteroscopy in patients with obscure gastrointestinal bleeding. Am J Gastroenterol. 2006;101:52–7.
35. Matsumoto T, Esaki M, Moriyama T, Nakamura S, Iida M. Comparison of capsule endoscopy and enteroscopy with the double-balloon method in patients with obscure bleeding and polyposis. Endoscopy. 2005;37:827–32.
36. Nakamura M, Niwa Y, Ohmiya N, et al. Preliminary comparison of capsule endoscopy and double-balloon enteroscopy in patients with suspected small-bowel bleeding. Endoscopy. 2006;38:59–66.
37. Matsumoto T, Moriyama T, Esaki M, Nakamura S, Iida M. Performance of antegrade double-balloon enteroscopy: comparison with push enteroscopy. Gastrointest Endosc. 2005;62:392–8.
38. Hayat M, Axon AT, O'Mahony S. Diagnostic yield and effect on clinical outcomes of push enteroscopy in suspected small-bowel bleeding. Endoscopy. 2000;32:369–72.
39. Nguyen NQ, Rayner CK, Schoeman MN. Push enteroscopy alters management in a majority of patients with obscure gastrointestinal bleeding. J Gastroenterol Hepatol. 2005;20:716–21.
40 Plum N, May AD, Manner H, Ell C. [Peutz–Jeghers syndrome: endoscopic detection and treatment of small bowel polyps by double-balloon enteroscopy]. Z Gastroenterol. 2007;45:1049–55.
41. Schwartz GD, Barkin JS. Small-bowel tumors detected by wireless capsule endoscopy. Dig Dis Sci. 2007;52:1026–30.

42. Hadithi M, Al-toma A, Oudejans J, van Bodegraven AA, Mulder CJ, Jacobs M. The value of double-balloon enteroscopy in patients with refractory celiac disease. Am J Gastroenterol. 2007;102:987–96.
43. Mensink P, Haringsma J, Kucharzik T et al. Complications of double balloon enteroscopy: a multicenter survey. Endoscopy. 2007;39:613–15.
44. Möschler O, May AD, Müller MK, Ell C; DBE-Studiengruppe Deutschland. [Complications in double-balloon enteroscopy: results of the German DBE registry]. Z Gastroenterol. 2008;46:266–70.

5
Bile duct system/papilla of Vater: standards and innovations

B. SCHUMACHER and H. NEUHAUS

DIAGNOSTIC

Biliary strictures can result from malignant or benign tumours and it is important that, if an endoscopic retrograde cholangiopancreatography (ERCP) is performed, maximal attempts are made to obtain a tissue diagnosis. Sensitivity of tissue sampling by brush cytology, fine-needle aspiration or forceps biopsy is quite low at about 51%; with a combination of all three techniques this will increase to 68%. Per-oral cholangioscopy, a technique that uses a fibreoptic cholangioscope passed through a therapeutic duodenoscope directly into the biliary tract, has been shown to improve the ability to distinguish malignant from benign biliary strictures. Filling defects seen on ERCP can be caused by various benign or malignant tumours and by bile duct stones. Only direct endoscopic visualization can diagnose those filling defects and undertake appropriate therapy; it has now been clearly established that this can improve accuracy in the diagnosis of biliary filling defects[1]. In this study 91 patients were evaluated; there were 76 strictures and 21 filling defects. Of the patients with filling defects ERCP alone was able to correctly identify eight malignant lesions and nine benign tumours, but ERCP did not correctly diagnose four cases of stone disease. Cholangioscopy using the direct cholangioscopic criteria for malignancy was tested in 76 patients, and improved the diagnostic accuracy for strictures to 93%[1].

In addition a German group confirmed these data in a study of 53 patients with primary sclerosing cholangitis (PSC). Cholangioscopy was performed to distinguish between benign and malignant dominant bile duct stenoses[2]. Twelve patients had dominant bile duct stenoses caused by cholangiocarcinoma, whereas 41 of 53 patients had benign dominant bile duct strictures. Cholangioscopy was superior to ERCP for detecting malignancy in terms of its sensitivity of 92% vs 66%, specificity of 93% vs 51% and accuracy of 93% vs 55%.

However, normal cholangioscopy has some disadvantages: two endoscopists are needed, and the system is very fragile with high repair costs. Spyglass is a newly developed per-oral cholangioscope system which allows a single-operator examination with a four-way deflectable steering tip. This new technology employs a single-use 10 Fr multi-channelled sheath that attaches to the head of the duodenoscope just below the biopsy port and advances through the accessory channel for insertion into the duct. The sheath provides steering of the tip, illumination, water flushing, a channel for passage of a 0.035 calibre fibreoptic probe for visualization of the duct (Spy Scope) and another for either wire guidance or passage of biopsy forceps (Figure 1).

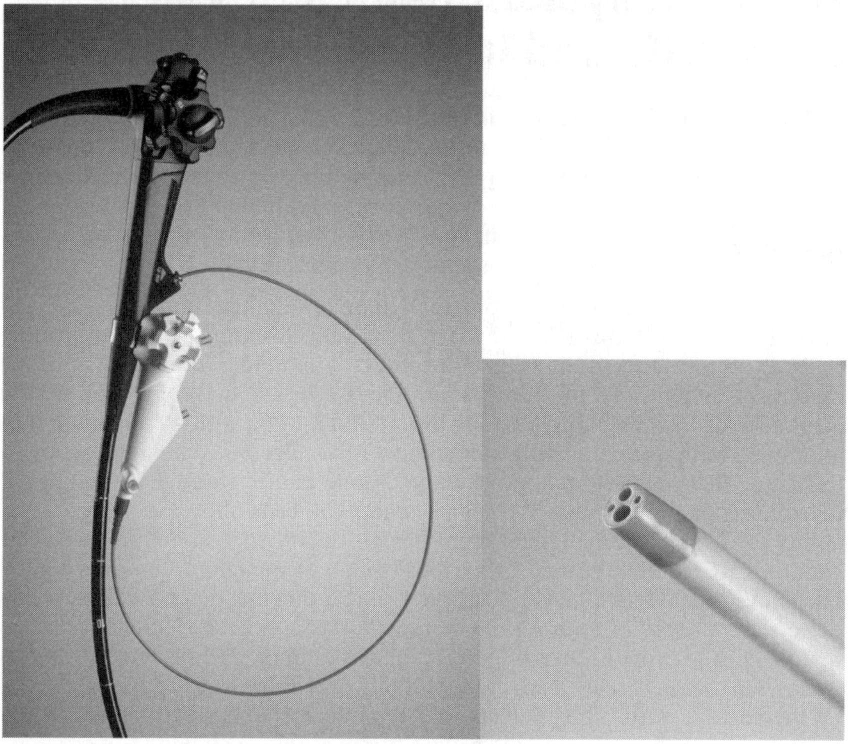

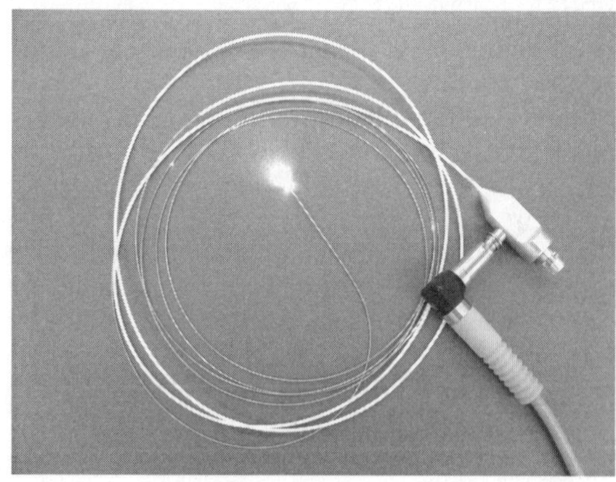

Figure 1 **A**: Spy-Glass direct visualization system attached to the duodenoscope and advanced into the accessory channel. **B**: Spy-Glass fibreoptic probe

In an international multicentre registry 146 patients were included. Indications for spyglass examinations were: indeterminate strictures non-PSC 39%, stone management 34%, suspected strictures in PSC 10%, indeterminate filling defects 6% and other 12%. The procedural success was 89% overall. Visual diagnosis was discordant from ERCP diagnosis in 21%. Concordance between visual diagnosis and biopsy results was 71%. All the procedures could safely be performed by one operator[3,4].

To improve the images of the fibreoptic cholangioscope a new endoscopic system based on narrowing the bandwidth of spectral transmittance of red–green–blue optical filters (NBI), was developed. This system may yield clear images of the surface structure and microvessels of the common bile duct. An article by Itoi et al.[5] describes a novel application of NBI in the bile duct. The authors used a newly developed 3.4 mm diameter cholangioscope that was passed through a duodenoscope to image the bile duct. This system uses two narrow-band filters (centred at 414 nm and 540 nm); optical magnification was not available. In this study 21 lesions were evaluated by using per-oral cholangioscopy with light imaging and NBI. Visualization of only two lesions was excellent by conventional observation, visualization by NBI was excellent in 12 lesions. NBI was equal to or better than white-light endoscopy in identifying both surface structure and mucosal vessels.

IDUS (intraductal ultrasonography), at the time of ERCP, may add useful information in patients with suspected pancreaticobiliary malignancy, especially cholangiocarcinoma. However, there are limited data and the exact role has not yet been defined.

IDUS has a high resolution because of the use of high-frequency ultrasound (20–30 Hz) and can be performed in a single session with ERCP because the IDUS probe can be inserted via the channel of a side-viewing duodenoscope. IDUS has a staging accuracy in patients with ampullary neoplasm ranging between 88% and 93%. Previously published data have shown correctly diagnosed ductal infiltration by IDUS in patients with ampullary neoplasm in 90%[6].

PSC

PSC is a chronic inflammatory disease of the biliary tree. It is characterized by stricturing and dilation of the intrahepatic and/or extrahepatic bile ducts. PSC is associated with an unpredictable risk of developing cholangiocarcinoma in up to 30%. PSC is diagnosed by radiographic imaging of the biliary tree, traditionally performed by using ERCP but more recently magnetic resonance cholangiopancreatography (MRCP) is thought to be as sensitive as ERCP in the diagnosis of PSC. The role of ERCP in the diagnosis of PSC has become controversial with the availability of high-quality MRCP, because several studies which have compared ERCP and MRCP in these patients have shown that MRCP has a comparable diagnostic accuracy. In a study with 150 patients with cholestatic liver enzymes 146 of these patients were studied by MRCP. PSC was found in 34 patients (23%) with ERCP, and MRCP was able to correctly identify 88% and had a specificity of 99%[7]. A similar study determined that MRCP had a diagnostic accuracy of 90% compared to 97% with invasive cholangiography in 73 patients. However, three-quarters of the PSC patients required therapeutic interventions[8]. ERCP is the first technique and still the gold standard. The endoscopic therapy is indicated if there is clinical evidence of cholangitis or if a dominant stricture is suspected. Balloon dilation and short-term (10–14-day) stenting is preferable.

A European study described 32 PSC patients with dominant strictures treated with plastic stent placement for a mean of only 11 days. Improvements in symptoms and cholestasis were seen in all patients, and these improvements were maintained for several years with 80% of patients intervention-free at 1 year and 60% at 3 years[9]. The addition of ursodeoxycholic acid (UDCA) to endoscopic therapy has been examined in a prospective trial in 106 PSC patients followed up for 13 years[10]. All patients received UDCA along with balloon dilation of dominant strictures or placement of short-term biliary stenting whenever necessary. The combined approach appeared to improve overall survival rates, but it was unclear whether the UDCA, the endoscopic therapy or the combination of the two treatments improved outcome.

Complications after therapeutic procedures in PSC patients are more frequent than after diagnostic ERCP. Factors that appeared to increase the risk of complications included a therapeutic indication such as jaundice or cholangitis. These patients had a 14% complication rate[11,12]. In a recently published study the investigators compared ERCP-related complications among patients with PSC with a control group with biliary stricture but no PSC. Complications after therapeutic ERCP were not increased among patients with PSC compared with patients with biliary strictures who do not have PSC. The overall complication rate was 12.9% after ERCP among patients with PSC[13].

Cholangiocarcinoma will develop in up to 10–30% of patients with PSC with a life-time risk of 10–15%. Early diagnosis may improve survival as it may permit curative surgical resection. Several endoscopic methods have been evaluated to diagnose cholangiocarcinoma in PSC. Brush cytology, fine-needle aspiration and forceps biopsy have low sensitivity and high specificity. Combining tumour markers with cytology may increase sensitivity[14,15].

BILIARY SPHINCTEROTOMY

Well-established indications for endoscopic sphincterotomy (EST) are common bile duct stones, acute cholangitis, palliation of ampullary malignancies and facilitation of biliary stent placement. The complication rate is reported to be 9.8%. Acute pancreatitis is the most frequent complication with 5.4%[16]. An alternative procedure to EST is balloon sphincteroplasty, especially in patients with coagulopathies and those in whom the endoscopic approach is difficult (duodenal diverticulum; BII anatomy). Compared to EST in a meta-analysis of several randomized studies, endoscopic balloon dilation (EBD) can cause less bleeding but a higher rate of post-ERCP pancreatitis (7.4% vs 4.3%)[17]. Another large prospective US multicentre study randomized EBD with EST for extraction of bile duct stones. The success rates were comparable but the overall morbidity (17.9% vs 3.3%) was significantly higher in patients who had undergone EBD[18]. Technical details of EBD may influence the clinical outcome. The problem is that this procedure has not yet been standardized in terms of inflation-pressure, time or number of inflations. The potential advantage of preserved sphincter function remains undetermined. Long-term data after EBD showed a higher frequency of stone recurrence compared to EST[19]. Based on these data EBD cannot be recommended as a routine procedure, but should be a valuable alternative in patients with a difficult endoscopic approach.

Long-term consequences of EST are cautery-induced distal bile duct strictures and development of bile duct stones. The overall rate of late symptoms ranges from 6% to 24%. A correlation between size of EST and late complications cannot be determined[20].

STENTS

In a patient with suspected malignant biliary obstruction the key decision is whether the patient is a candidate for curative resection. This is based on the patient's age and medical condition, because aggressive resection is appropriate. If a patient is not resectable, palliative stenting for relief of jaundice, pruritus and improvement of life quality should be performed. The use of plastic stents has been plagued by early occlusion requiring replacement every 3–4 months. As a result of the deficiencies of plastic stents, self-expanding metal stents (SEMS) were developed to relieve malignant obstruction without the need for repeat intervention. Randomized studies comparing SEMS to plastic demonstrated longer patency rates and decreased rates of cholangitis[21–23]. The median patency for metal stents is approximately double that for plastic stents, and the overall cost is substantially lower for metal stents because of fewer reinterventions. However, a 19–40% occlusion rate of metal stents has been observed in several studies[22,23]. Occluded SEMS are managed by insertion of a plastic stent within the occluded SEMS, insertion of a second SEMS or by mechanical cleaning of the occluded lumen. Recently, a covered SEMS was developed to reduce occlusion induced by tissue ingrowths. Covered SEMS provide the size advantage of uncovered SEMS with the promise of prevention of tissue ingrowths through the interstices of the metal mesh and the prospect of removability. The potential of durable patency and removability make covered SEMS an attractive option for endoluminal therapy of malignant and benign strictures.

However, in comparative coated SEMS studies, statistically significant reductions in occlusion and patency rates have not been demonstrated. Additionally the results showed a trend towards a higher incidence of complications including pancreatitis, cholecystitis and migration[24–26].

Hilar tumours have proven to be a challenge to treat and manage because of their poor sensitivity to conventional therapies. All patients should be fully evaluated for resectability before any type of intervention. If a patient is not resectable endoscopic stent drainage has been proposed as an alternative palliative treatment. Hilar tumours are often problematic for ERCP. MRCP

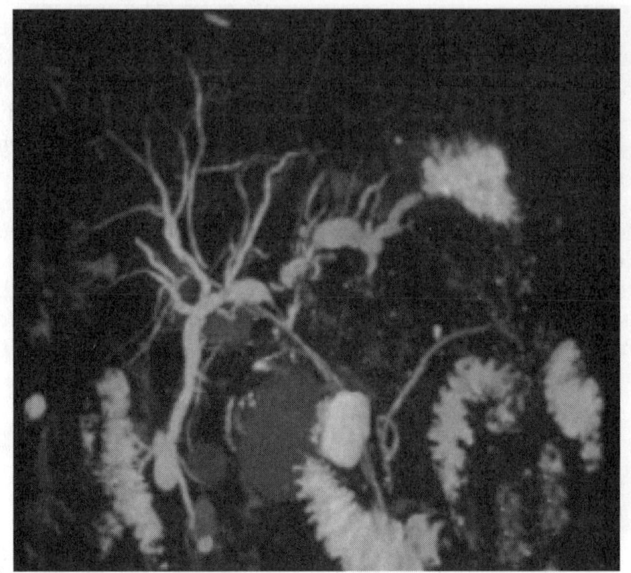

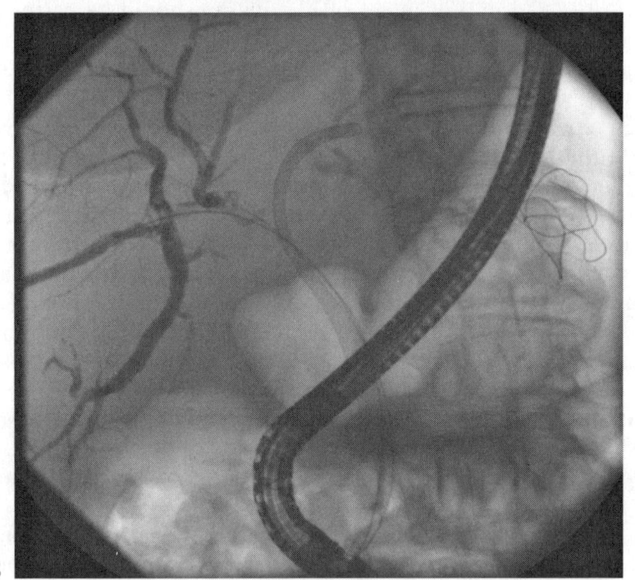

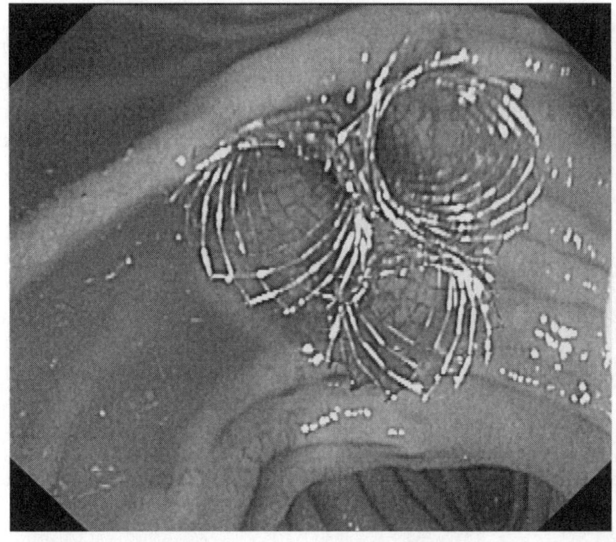

Figure 2 (and opposite)   **A**: Patient with Klatskin tumour: MRCP shows dilation of segment V and III. **B**: Selective guidewire insertion of the stenotic segments and implantation of metal stents. **C**: Endoscopic view of the implantated metal stents

should be performed earlier, because it is very accurate at staging the extent of the tumour without risk of cholangitis[27].

The technique of stent implantation includes several options: draining only one system; draining both systems; and which stent material to use. In patients who have complex strictures (Bismuth IV) the central question is whether adequate palliative relief of obstruction requires placement of two endoprostheses, or if placing one will be sufficient. The necessity to ensure the drainage of both systems, including additional endoscopic or percutaneous stent, pertains more to the prevention of procedure-induced cholangitis caused by contrast injection in undrained biliary branches than to effective palliation. Generally, if both lobes are imaged with contrast, bilateral stenting reduces the potential sequelae of cholangitis in contaminated but undrained areas. If contrast does not contaminate both sides then unilateral stenting should be sufficient[28]. In a prospective study of 61 patients with hilar strictures, unilateral stent placement was achieved in 97%; jaundice resolved in 86.9%. Cholangitis developed in three patients within the first week[29]. MRCP can involve selective drainage with metal stents. If there is one dominant side identified by MRCP then selective cannulation with a catheter and a guidewire should be attempted and a single stent can be placed. Bilateral SEMS may be placed alongside one another, or the second may be deployed through the mesh of the initial SEMS. Two guidewires are used to maintain access to the right and left biliary systems while placing bilateral stents. Sometimes it can be difficult to place the second stent beside the first stent. In one study it was demonstrated that the placement of a temporary plastic stent in the common bile duct (CBD) prevents the full expansion of the first stent to facilitate placement of the second SEMS[30.]

Metal stents should result in better drainage than plastic stents in hilar strictures because metal stents do not occlude side-branches and stent patency is longer than in plastic stents. In contrast to plastic stents, metal ones are not removable after the first few days of deployment. Thus metal stents should be used in patients with proven unresectable malignancies.

The goal of best palliative therapy in hilar tumours should be: (a) MRCP as the first diagnostic procedure; (b) draining of the stenotic segments as thoroughly as possible by ERCP or percutaneous transhepatic cholangioscopic drainage (PTCD); (c) drainage using non-covered SEMS.

References

1. Fukuda Y, Tsuyuguchi T, Sakai Y et al. Diagnostic utility of peroral cholangioscopy for various bile duct lesions. Gastrointest Endosc. 2005;62:374–82.
2. Tischendorf JJW, Krüger M, Trautwein C et al. Cholangioscopic characterization of dominant bile duct stenoses in patients with primary sclerosing cholangitis. Endoscopy. 2006;38 665–9.
3. Cheng YK, Parsi MA, Binmoeller K et al. Peroral cholangioscopy (PO) using a disposable steerable single operator catheter for biliary stone therapy and assessment of interdeterminate strictures: a multi-center experience using Spy-Glass. Gastrointest Endosc. 2008;67:no.5 (abstract 103).
4. Chen YK, Pleskow DK. Spy-Glass single-operator peroral cholangiopancreatoscopy system for the diagnosis and therapy of bile-duct disorders: a clinical feasibility study. Gastrointest Endosc. 2007;65:832–41.
5. Itoi T, Sofuni A, Itokawa F et al. Peroral cholangioscopic diagnosis of biliary-tract diseases by using narrow-band imaging. Gastrointest Endosc. 2007;66:730–6.
6. Ito K, Fuyita N, Noda Y et al. Preoperative evaluation of ampullary neoplasm with EUS and transpapillary intraductal US: a prospective and histopathologically controlled study. Gastrointest Endosc. 2007;66:740–7.
7. Textor HJ, Flacke S, Pauleit D et al. Three-dimensional magnetic resonance cholangiography with respiratory triggering in the diagnosis of primary sclerosing cholangitis: comparison with endoscopic retrograde cholangiography. Endoscopy. 2002;34:984–90.
8. Angulo P, Pearce DH, Johnson CD et al. Magnetic resonance cholangiography in patients with biliary disease: its role in primary sclerosing cholangitis. J Hepatol. 2000;33:520–7.
9. Ponsioen CY, Lam K, van Milligen de Wit et al. Four years experience with short term stenting in primary sclerosing cholangitis. Am J Gastroenterol. 1999;94:2403–7.
10. Stiehl A, Rudolph G, Kloters-Plachky P et al. Development of dominant bile duct stenoses in patients with primary sclerosing cholangitis treated with ursodeoxycholic acid: outcome after endoscopic treatment. J Hepatol. 2002;36:151–6.
11. Bjornsson E, Lindquist-Ottosson J, Asztely M et al. Dominant strictures in patients with primary sclerosing cholangitis. Am J Gastroenterol. 2004;99:502–8.
12. Baluyut AR, Sherman S, Lehman GA et al. Impact of endoscopic therapy on the survival of patients with primary sclerosing cholangitis. Gastrointest Endosc. 2001;53:308–12.
13. Etzel J, Eng S, Ko C et al. Complications after ERCP in patients with primary sclerosing cholangitis. Gastrointest Endosc. 2008;67:643–50.
14. Khalid A, Pal R, Sasatomi E et al. Use of microsatellite marker loss of heterozygosity in accurate diagnosis of pancreatico biliary malignancy from brush cytology samples. Gut. 2004;53:1860–5.
15. Baron TH, Harewood GC, Rumalla A et al. A prospective comparison of digital image analysis and routine cytology for the identification of malignancy in biliary tract strictures. Clin Gastroenterol Hepatol. 2004;2:214–19.
16. Masci E, Toti G, Mariani A et al. Complications of diagnostic and therapeutic ERCP: a prospective multicenter study. Am J Gastroenterol. 2001;96:417–23.

17. Baron TH, Harewood GC. Endoscopic balloon dilation of the biliary sphincter compared to endoscopic biliary sphincterotomy for removal of bile duct stones during ERCP: a metaanalysis of randomized,controlled trials. Am J Gastroenterol. 2004;99:1455–60.

18. Di Sario JA, Freeman ML, Bjorkman DJ et al. Endoscopic balloon dilation compared with sphincterotomy for extraction of bile duct stones. Gastroenterology. 2004;127:1291–9.

19. Tanaka S, Sawayama T, Yoshioka T. Endoscopic papillary balloon dilation and endoscopic sphincterotomy for bile duct stones: long term outcomes in a prospective randomized controlled trial. Gastrointest Endosc. 2004;59:614–18.

20. Prat F. The long term consequence of endoscopic sphincterotomy. Acta Gastro-Enterol Belg. 2000;63:395–6.

21. Davids PH, Groen AK, Rauws EA et al. Randomized trial of self-expanding metal stents versus polyethylene stents for distal malignant biliary obstruction. Lancet. 1992;340:1488–92.

22. Knyrim K, Wagner HJ, Pausch J et al. A prospective, randomized, controlled trial of metal stents for malignant obstruction of the common bile duct. Endoscopy. 1993;25:207–12.

23. Kaassis M, Boyer J, Dumas R et al. Plastic or metal stents for malignant stricture of the common bile duct? Results of a randomized prospective study. Gastrointest Endosc. 2003;57:178–82.

24. Fumex F, Coumaros D, Napoleon B et al. Similar performance but higher cholecystitis rate with covered biliary stents: results from a prospective multicenter evaluation. Endoscopy. 2006;38:787–92.

25. Yoon WJ, Lee JK,Lee KH et al. A comparison of covered and uncovered Wallstents for the management of distal malignant biliary obstruction. Gastrointest Endosc. 2006;63:996–1000.

26. Park do H, Kim MH, Choi JS et al. Covered vs uncovered Wallstents for malignant extrahepatic biliary obstruction: a cohort comparative analysis. Clin Gastroenterol Hepatol. 2006;4:190–6.

27. Hintze RE, Abou-Rebyek H, Adler A et al. Magnetic resonance cholangio-pancreatography-guided unilateral endoscopic stent placement for Klatskin tumors. Gastrointest Endosc. 2001;53:40–6.

28. ASGE guideline: The role of ERCP in diseases of the biliary tract and the pancreas. Gastrointest Endosc. 2001;53:40–6.

29. Deviere J, Baize M, de Toeuf J et al. Long-term follow-up of patients with hilar malignant strictures treated by endoscopic internal biliary drainage. Gastrointest Endosc. 1988;34:95–101.

30. Hookey LC, Le Moine O, Deviere J. Use of a temporary plastic stent to facilitate the placement of multiple self-expanding metal stents in malignant biliary hilar strictures. Gastrointest Endosc. 2005;62:605–9.

Section IV
Endosonography

Chair: C MEYENBERGER and M JUNG

6
Endoscopic ultrasound: overview

C. F. DIETRICH and A. P. BARREIROS

INTRODUCTION

Diagnostic and therapeutic endoscopic ultrasound (EUS) has become an essential endoscopic procedure as it provides the unique option of evaluating the luminal and extraluminal features of the gastrointestinal tract. Within the oesophagus, stomach and rectum obvious clinical issues are answered by EUS, leading to therapeutic consequences and individual therapeutic decisions. In an even more complex manner, EUS is performed for the evaluation of additional organs such as pancreas or adrenal glands. Furthermore, EUS is an invaluable tool at the intersection of multiple medical disciplines leading to an interdisciplinary approach in favour of the patient (e.g. gastroenterology and pneumology concerning the mediastinum, gastroenterology and endocrinology regarding adrenal glands or gastroenterology and surgery within minimal invasive interventions).

On the basis of several organ systems and tumours, this chapter covers the variety of current diagnostic and therapeutic options of EUS.

TECHNIQUES

Generally, linear EUS scopes and scanners are most commonly used due to the option of performing interventions and biopsies besides diagnostic approaches. Nevertheless, most published studies evaluating the upper gastrointestinal (GI) tract were performed with radial scopes[1,2]. Mini-probes ultrasound is commonly used to evaluate the layers of the GI tract in a more precise manner due to their high spatial resolution, using up to 30 MHz frequency. However, an intraductal mini-probes technique is performed by a few centres only. Within recent years only target therapeutic EUS techniques were evaluated in mostly monocentric surveillance studies. Therefore, the validity of these studies remains questionable.

The goal of all imaging techniques, including EUS, is to detect but also to characterize pathological findings. To succeed, a variety of different techniques are applied. Evaluation of tissue elasticity is a main component of endoscopy ('endopalpation') and sonography ('sonopalpation') and may now also be displayed colour-coded. Colour-coded duplex ultrasound (vascularization, vessel anatomy) and elastography (consistency, texture) allow an optimal integral examination technique, targeted punctures and in particular avoidance of complications. Contrast-enhanced endosonography is not yet generally established[3] but this technique allows to visualize small and minimal vessels (vascularization pattern) and shows promising preliminary results, particularly in the differential diagnosis of pancreatic lesions when performed by an experienced investigator.

Note 1: Colour-coded duplex ultrasound is an integral part of endosonographic examination techniques evaluating the upper and lower gastrointestinal tract even if there is a lack of prospective studies focusing on the benefit of this technique. The personal assessment for elastography of the author is similar even if this method is up to now offered by only one company.

COMPARISON OF METHODS AND EXAMINATION TECHNIQUES

The radial echoendoscope technique is comparable to a cross-section of computed tomography (CT) or magnetic resonance imaging (MRI). It displays the layers of the oesophagus precisely. In contrast, longitudinal EUS is similar to transabdominal ultrasound and comprises the unique option of intervention. In the authors' opinion most clinical questions can be answered appropriately and investigated with a longitudinal sector scanner, although numerous studies cited in this chapter were performed using radial echoendoscope technique. The group of Thomas Rösch must be granted credit for performing several endosonographic studies with radial EUS. Radial (rigid) probes do have both diagnostic and therapeutic advantages in the anorectal region and must therefore be considered the standard technique. High-resolution (radial) mini-probes with high ultrasound frequency (up to 30 MHz) are able to visualize the mucosa and submucosa of the upper and lower GI tract, as well as to differentiate the papillary region, and were also conceived/designed for intraductal biliopancreatic duct analysis.

EUS-GUIDED FINE-NEEDLE ASPIRATION (EUS-FNA) TECHNIQUE

A variety of different FNA techniques were described in the literature, although large studies are still missing. From the available literature the following conclusions may be drawn: the needle diameter should be chosen as small as possible and at the same time still effective for puncture and extraction of cytology (22G, optionally 25G). When tissue is obtained, it should be fixed in formalin before histological processing. With commonly used puncture needles histological tissue examinations are not routinely possible even if several authors have published promising results. Currently available rigid-needle systems for obtaining histological tissue probes, in particular for puncture of the pancreatic head, still require further development with respect to a more variable needle guidance. Indications for fine needle aspiration cytology are summarized in Table 1.

Table 1 Indications for fine-needle-aspiration-cytology

Documentation of malignancy in patients with unresectable pancreatic tumour before palliative therapy
To exclude other tumour entities
In patients who hesitate as regards undergoing a radical operation technique, due to a relatively high mortality
Documentation of benignity in low pre-test chance for a malignant mass

COMPLICATIONS OF EUS

Complications of EUS were reported predominantly in casuistic notes, retrospective analyses, case series or surveys[4,5]. It has to be distinguished between examinations performed using orthograd scopes or side-view scopes with a device-specific variability (rigidity of the tip) and complications due to interventions.

Typical complications are perforations, aspirations and bacteraemia. A European multicentre study analysing complications in radial EUS technique described 13/37 915 (0.03%) perforations of the oesophagus. Similar results were reported in a survey performed in the USA in 2001, reporting 16/43 852 (0.03%) perforations of the cervical oesophagus (two patients underwent surgery, one patient died).

Risk factors are oesophagus carcinoma as well as a dilation of a malignant stenosis of the oesophagus, advanced age of the patient, degenerative vertebral column variances, an inexperienced examiner, as well as a complicated introduction of the scope due to previous endoscopic examinations.

Note 2: Diagnostic EUS is a secure procedure with complications comparable to other diagnostic endoscopic examinations of the upper GI tract. Most frequent complications are perforations of the oesophagus or duodenum, preferentiated by specific and optical properties of the echoendoscopes.

COMPLICATIONS DUE TO ENDOSONOGRAPHIC INTERVENTIONS

Performing interventions, a significantly higher risk of complications has been reported compared to solely diagnostic examinations. Complications may be bleedings, infections and tumour cell seeding, when interventions are performed on cystic lesions, as well as acute pancreatitis.

Self-limiting minor intraluminal and extraluminal bleedings were observed in individual patients. The risk of bleeding during puncture of cystic lesions is higher. Acetylsalicyl acid or non-steroidal antiphlogistics and low-molecular weight heparin does increase the risk. One lethal bleeding after endosonographic FNA of a pancreatic pseudoaneurysm using a radial technique without colour-coded duplex analysis was published. Therefore, colour-coded duplex analysis to identify local blood vessels before puncture is indispensable.

There is a significant risk of infections when performing EUS-FNA of cystic lesions of the pancreas and particularly in the mediastinum. Prophylactic treatment with antibiotics is obligatory before EUS-FNA of cystic lesions, even if all published studies are historically comparisons between punctures performed with or without prophylactic antibiotic treatment.

Performing endosonography in patients with chronic pancreatitis, retroperitoneal infections were reported in 3/167 (1.8%) of all patients, after blockade of the ganglion coeliacum (plexus neurolysis, EUS-celiac plexus block/neurolysis (CPB)). Application of this technique in pancreatic tumours means less, but still considerable risk of, infections.

EUS-FNA of colorectal tumours using transrectal and transcolic punctures of adjacent lesions seems to be secure despite microbial contamination of the gastrointestinal lumen. Only one patient has been described so far suffering from an infectious complication after EUS-FNA of a pelvic lesion.

Several case reports of needle tract metastasis after EUS-FNA of pancreatic carcinoma or lymph node metastasis of malignant melanoma were published. In addition, peritoneal seeding after EUS-FNA of a malignant intraductal papillary mucinous pancreatic neoplasia (IPMN) was also documented. However, at present no systematically collected data are available.

The incidence of post-interventional acute pancreatitis was reported to be between 0.29% and 2.0%. It is noteworthy that in 50% of all patients suffering from acute pancreatitis after EUS-FNA a benign pancreatic disease was diagnosed. The rate of complications in EUS-CPB and EUS-guided pancreatogastrostomy must be assumed to be higher.

Note 3: The overall complications of EUS-FNA are – depending on the indication and documentation form of complications – between 0.3% and 6.3%.

PREVENTION OF COMPLICATIONS

Strategies to avoid or reduce potential complications, and in particular to evaluate the potential benefit for patients with co-morbidity, as well as to determine the ideal setting for planned endosonographic interventions, should be known by the examiner. An endoscopic examination with orthograd optic should be performed before EUS examination with a side-view scope to exclude a stenosis. In case of EUS-FNA or EUS-guided drainage of cystic lesions (pancreas, peripancreatic, mediastinal) peri-interventional treatment with antibiotics is recommended. Finally appropriate and extensive training is also essential to reduce the risk of these examinations.

CARCINOMA OF THE OESOPHAGUS

Preoperative staging of oesophagus carcinoma was among the first applications of endosonography since 1980. It offers a high diagnostic specificity of infiltration (T-stadium) of the neoplasia. In published studies with more than 100 patients an accuracy of 80–95% was demonstrated. However, the specificity in T1 and T2 tumours was lower than in T3 or T4 carcinoma, although prospective data analysing this question are sparsely published.

Earlier published data showed that EUS tended to overestimate the tumour stage due to peritumoral inflammation. The results of accurate lymph node staging are even lower (65–85%), since lymph nodes may be infiltrated independently of their size in a circumscribed manner. Furthermore a relevant interobserver variability was published[6].

The aim of all preoperative diagnostic examinations in oesophageal carcinoma is to identify patients in whom curative R0 resection is possible (criteria: circumscribed depth of infiltration ($\leqslant$T2), exclusion of lymph nodes and metastasis (N0, M0).

Note 4: Detection of a carcinoma of the oesophagus makes endosonography obligatory. Exceptions: high-grade stenosis; re-staging.

Due to significant morbidity and mortality in thoraco-abdominal resection of the oesophagus, patients with an early carcinoma (T1m) and prognostic relevant co-morbidities may also undergo endoscopic therapy with a curative intention (endoscopic mucosa resection, EMR). This minimal invasive technique may only be used if the tumour does not infiltrate the submucosa. The differentiation of mucosal infiltration can be achieved endosono-graphically with high specificity[7].

Endosonographic options for the differentiation of mucosal and submucosal infiltration of tumours are highly controversial in the literature[8]. However, prospective multicentre-collected data comparing conventional radial endosonography with mini-probe technology in a non-selected population, in order to distinguish on submucosal infiltration of a tumour, are lacking.

A German monocentre study analysing the application of endosonography using mini-probes to differentiate T1m and T1sm stadium, could surprisingly not show the expected advantage over standard EUS[8]. To the contrary, Japanese studies found that the extension of submucosal infiltration (analysed in thirds) was identified correctly[9]. This is of major interest because tumours infiltrating deep submucosal layers have a significantly higher rate of malignant lymph node infiltration.

It is not feasible to perform a R0 resection in an advanced stage of squamous cell carcinoma. If tumour growth exceeds the oesophagus wall with or without lymph node metastasis (N+) and after exclusion of distant metastasis (M0) neoadjuvant therapy modalities are used as an attempt to reduce tumour mass, eradicate micrometastasis and improve outcome after resection of a local advanced squamous cell carcinoma of the oesophagus. With neoadjuvant therapy median survival could be prolonged and a reduction of local recurrence was achieved in 20%.

Endosonography is also first choice in the examination and evaluation of mural exceeding growth in contrast to a lack of sufficiency in *exclusion* of lymph node metastasis. Furthermore, endosonography is the first choice to examine lymph nodes adjacent to the truncus coeliacus. In this setting EUS is superior to all other imaging techniques. EUS-FNA with cytological analysis of lymph nodes has increased diagnostic options in positive EUS findings.

However, in case of negative cytological results from FNA this may not be considered reliable.

OPEN QUESTIONS ON STAGING OF LYMPH NODES

In 1986, Tio and Tytgat specified criteria for a definition of 'normal' and 'metastatic' modified lymph nodes in endosonographic examination. They described specific criteria such as size (>6–10 mm), echopoor texture, round form and sharp margin. All these criteria have a high interobserver variability. Early published data generated an accuracy of up to 85%. Current data show inferior results and do not allow a reliable determination of the dignity.

OPEN QUESTION ON DETECTION OF RECURRENT DISEASE

After R0 resection of the oesophagus almost 50% of patients develop a local recurrence of the disease or distant metastases. In these patients endosonography may be helpful when they present with recurrent symptoms during follow-up and an irregular, echopoor mural thickening. For this specific application the sensitivity of EUS is higher than 75%. However, regular layering is abrogated in the area of the anastomosis; thus in asymptomatic patients endosonography may be prone to false-positive results (with washy layers). In contrast, for focal mural thickening or a tumour next to the oesophageal wall or stomach, EUS has a positive predictive value up to 100% for recurrent disease.

STOMACH

Carcinoma of the stomach

Similar to the oesophageal setting in gastric lesions EUS provides on the one hand the necessary security prior to endoscopic resection (exact determination of infiltration, exclusion of metastases of the lymph nodes) and on the other hand a correct evaluation of a T3 and/or N+ stadium, implicating a neoadjuvant therapy. T2 tumours may be overestimated due to limited identifiability of the serosa. With respect to T-stage and evaluation of regional lymph nodes or metastases, EUS is superior to other imaging procedures such as computed tomography (CT), magnetic resonance imaging (MRI) and positron emission tomography (PET), particularly in combination with fine-needle aspiration (EUS-FNA). It remains unclear whether EUS mini-probe technology is superior to conventional radial or longitudinal endosonography techniques.

> *Note 5*: With detection of a stomach carcinoma endosonography is obligatory, on the one hand, to recognize local tumour stage with the necessary accuracy before endoscopic resection, and on the other hand to determine a neoadjuvant situation correctly.

GASTROINTESTINAL LYMPHOMA

Decisions on necessary diagnostic and therapeutic procedures and prognosis are dependent on an accurate histological classification and grading (low malignancy, secondarily high malignancy, high malignancy), stage of the lymphoma and localization.

The primary diagnosis of a gastrointestinal lymphoma is followed by staging examinations, aiming to detect the dissemination of the disease. Staging is usually performed in accordance with the Ann Arbor classification in their modification after Musshoff, considering the differentiation of stage I after Radaszkiewicz.

The endosonographic appearance of the gastric lymphoma is variable, depending on its circumscriptive or diffuse growth. An infiltration of the mucosa and submucosa marks stage I1 and/or T1 N0 M0 and an additional infiltration of the muscularis propria without penetration of the subserosa stage I2, respectively T2 N0 M0. An infiltration of all wall layers with penetration of the serosa marks stages I2, respectively T3, an infiltration of neighbouring organs or fabric stage I2, respectively T4, and an infestation of perigastral lymph nodes stage II1 respectively T1-4N1.

The distinction of stages I and II in stage I1, I2 and II1 was proven to be prognostically relevant[10] and can be performed only with the help of endosonography, a unique imaging procedure for the differentiation of the gastric wall layers and also detection of perigastral lymphomas. Therefore it must nowadays be regarded as a routine investigation.

The diagnostic accuracy of preoperative EUS was evaluated in a large patient collective with the optimum gold standard of surgical preparation and histology[11], since all patients in this study with stomach lymphoma stages I and II underwent surgery. A correct endosonographic estimation in a multicentre study with 34 centres was possible in only 37 of 70 patients (53%).

Sensitivity for determination of the depth infiltration was 59% and lymph node status 71%. During the learning phase of EUS in this study, results were at first sight disappointing. With improved technologies (FNA, elastography) and increasing experience the results must be assumed to have increased lately. However, a proof for this hypothesis may no longer be obtained, due to the currently favoured conservative therapy in stomach lymphoma.

Subepithelial lesions

Reliable data on the incidence of subepithelial tumours and other subepithelial lesions of the digestive tract are missing, since the predominant group remains asymptomatic for life, and thus undiscovered. Although in autopsy studies mesenchymal tumours of the oesophagus (leiomyoma) are found with a frequency of 5%, and mesenchymal tumours in the stomach even age-dependent of up to 50%, clinically relevant subepithelial tumours are rare and mostly incidental findings (frequency distribution: stomach (60%), oesophagus (30%) and duodenum (10%)[12–14]).

In our own series 132/150 (88%) 105/125 (84%) of subepithelial tumours were random findings. A subepithelial tumour as a cause of any symptom (gastrointestinal bleeding, dysphagia or stenosis) is still rare. Endoscopy, just as radiological methods, is not sufficiently specific in the differentiation between subepithelial tumours, intramural varices and extraluminal impressions, as well as for the diagnosis of the nature of a tumour, its expansion, infiltration in neighbouring organs and depth localization within the wall of the gastrointestinal hollow organ. Thus, endosonography is the method of the choice for diagnosis of subepithelial tumours.

Note 6: EUS in a unique way permits description of the gastrointestinal wall layers and is thus superior to all other imaging procedures for the clarification of subepithelial lesions.

The role of EUS in diagnostics is particularly the description of the findings. The variety of echopoor subepithelial tumours is too large to make a definite diagnosis on a certain nosological entity depending solely on the endosonographic findings. The inclusion of anatomical predilections, as well as consideration of endosonographic details (layer allocation, outline/contour) leads to an improvement of the diagnostic descriptive options. On the basis of endosonographic criteria it should to be possible to make statements on the dignity of a tumour and to estimate the further diagnostic and therapeutic possibilities correctly. However, deviations from the typical findings may lead to errors.

Description and classification of subepithelial lesions by endosonography

The endosonographic description and classification of subepithelial tumours is based on the description of the definite localization (topography and affiliation to the layers), size (diameter in two levels standing perpendicularly one on the other), form, definability (sharply, in a diffuse way), delimitation (smoothly/ irregularly), allocation to the origin layer (possible/not possible, extramural), definability to adjacent layers, infiltration of extramural structures, malignancy (echofree, echogene, echopoor, mixed echogene) and internal texture, compressibility (by the probe, elastography), vascularity, and the detection of pathological loco regional lymph nodes (Table 2).

Endosonographic diagnosis of subepithelial tumours is subject to numerous subjective assessments and experience of the investigator. While the concordance among ten experienced investigators for cystic lesions (kappa 0.80) and extrinsic compressions was excellent (kappa 0.94) and good for lipoma (kappa 0.65), the degree of concordance was lower in the evaluation of leiomyoma (kappa 0.53) and vascular structures (kappa 0.54). The concordance in the evaluation of endosonographic dignity criteria ranged between unsatisfactory (cystic or echogene internal texture) to moderately good (heterogeneity, outline irregularity)[15] in the only published investigation.

Table 2 Classification of subepithelial lesions, modified by K. Hizawa et al.[16]

Vascular
   Varices
   Vascular malformations and haemangioma

Cystic
   Single-cystic (solitaire or multiple cysts)
   Polycystic or septated cystic
   Solid-cystic

Solid
   Echogenous (homogeneous, heterogeneous or inhomogenous)
   Echopoor (homogeneous, heterogeneous or inhomogenous)
   Mixed echogenicity (heterogeneous)

Numerous examiners tried to correlate different histopathological entities of subepithelial lesions with certain sonomorphological findings (Table 2).

The echofree subepithelial lesions may be divided into epithelialized cysts and pseudo cysts; the genuine mural cyst in the gastrointestinal tract is rarely observed and the underlying entity is manifold. The definite endosonographic classification of a cyst and/or a cystic lesion is not sufficiently reliable so that, as a primary goal of the endosonographic classification, the allocation of the dignity and the exact diagnostic and therapeutic procedure must be determined. Typically smoothly outlined echorich lipoma demarcates within the third (echogen) layer and is the most frequent echogene subepithelial lesion.

Note 7: The asymptomatic typical lipoma does not require further diagnostic and therapeutic examinations.

The spectrum of the very heterogeneous group of echopoor lesions comprises numerous benign tumours such as leiomyoma, granular cell tumours, neurinoma and inflammatory fibroid polyps (IFP), in addition, the relatively frequent benign and malignant gastrointestinal stroma tumours (GIST) (Table 3), neuroendocrine tumours, leiomyosarcoma and subepithelial metastases.

Table 3 Prognostic criteria of gastrointestinal stroma tumours[17]

Risk of malignant behaviour	Tumour size (cm)	Number of mitoses per HPF
Very low risk	<2	<5/50
Low risk	2–5	<5/50
Intermediate risk	<5	6–10/50
	5–10	<5/50
High risk	>5	>5/50
	>10	Any mitotic rate
	Any size	>10/50

Note 8: Attempts at endosonographic differentiation of echopoor subepithelial lesions, in particular the differentiation between GIST and leiomyoma, are not reliable.

The estimation of the malignancy risk of GIST is essentially based on the evaluation of the tumour size and number of mitoses per 50 high-power fields (HPF). Only tumours <(3 cm to) 5 cm and a low number of mitoses (<5/50 HPF) have a low risk of metastasis. The risk of metastasis of GIST depends on the anatomical localization: it is lower in gastric localizations compared to mesenteric localizations.

The correct estimation of the dignity of mesenchymal tumours of the digestive tract is more difficult compared to forceps biopsy-accessible epithelial neoplasia. The partially diverse data in the literature may be explained by a relatively small case number, a variety in the follow-up and the non-uniform handling of the term 'high-power field'.

In summary, criteria of benign subepithelial lesions were a tumour size up to 30 mm (in the lower gastrointestinal tract up to 20 mm), smooth outer contour, even echo sample without cystic texture, clear layer allocation, no signs of infiltration, no proof of suspect locoregional lymph nodes as well as in the follow-up: no significant size increase (for example >10 mm or 50%), no texture change and no new symptomatology, referred to the tumour (tumours with these criteria are classified as 'probably benign lesions').

Subepithelial tumours with a diameter of <30 mm, smooth outline and homogeneous texture were found to be always benign in a histological controlled endosonographic investigation of 56 subepithelial gastrointestinal mesenchymal tumours. However, at least one of these criteria was lacking in 63% of the benign mesenchymal tumours in the gastrointestinal tract[19]. There are published case reports of mesenchymal tumours of the digestive tract, following a clinically malignant course (in particular late hepatic metastasis and intraperitoneal dissemination), despite a benign characterization.

In larger histological controlled endosonographic studies a diameter >30 (–40) mm, irregular outer contour, heterogeneous internal structures and the rare proof of suspect local lymph nodes were typical for malignant biological behaviour.

The endoscopic (partial) resection of subepithelial tumours is the most effective strategy in order to obtain a safe histopathological diagnosis. In case of a high surgery risk and/or missing desire of the patient for an operation, a EUS-guided FNA may be an option.

Note 9: Endosonographic guided biopsy (EUS-FNA, EUS-TCB) of subepithelial lesions is poorly standardized, even though criteria for determination of the malignancy risk are defined.

Algorithm

After endosonographic exclusion of an extramural impression (up to 25% of the EUS indications) and of varices (<5%), which can simulate a subepithelial tumour, a lipoma is excluded (criteria: isoechogenous compared to the submucosa, more echogenous than muscularis propria (about 10% of the indications)). No further examinations are necessary. Similarly, this is valid in solitary (monocystic), echofree lesions without solidly (neoplastic) parts (highly likely benign). All other subepithelial lesions are analysed according to a standardized pattern.

Subepithelial tumours causing symptoms (bleeding, pain, stenosis symptomatic, endocrine activity), are always an indication for either endoscopic or surgical therapy.

Endoscopic and surgical options of resection are evaluated by EUS (tumour topography, depth infiltration and for the possible presence of suspect lymph nodes). An endoscopic resection is possible, if the tumour is <20 mm (maximally 30 mm with favourable localization) and separates well from the muscularis propria.

Note 10: A subepithelial lesion with corresponding pathology is always an indication for therapy.

In asymptomatic subepithelial tumours endosonography has the task to differentiate between:

- Lesions without the necessity for therapy or a follow-up (lipoma, typical (epithelial) benign cyst) with a high accuracy.

- Probably benign lesion which should undergo an endoscopic therapy or a follow-up at defined intervals.

- Potentially malignant tumours which may undergo endoscopic or surgical therapy (at least two endosonographic criteria referring to malignancy, significant increase of tumour size (>10 mm or 50%), changes of texture).

- Definitive malignant (for example infiltrating growing) or with high probability malignant tumours, for which only a surgical therapy is applicable.

Follow-up for benign lesions should be performed 6 months after initial diagnosis, after 1 year and after 2 years. Additional follow-up does not seem to be necessary for stable lesions. The main problems of endosonographic follow-up are costs and the insufficient compliance of patients.

HEPATOBILIARY SYSTEM

Cholelithiasis

Endosonography is the method of choice to exclude choledocholithiasis. The results of endosonography are independent of stone size and bile duct diameter, so that stones <2 mm can be visualized even in dilated bile ducts. However, a large prospective multicentre study proving the accuracy of EUS for the diagnostics of choledocholithiasis prior to cholecystectomy is still lacking.

The ERC(P) and endoscopic sphincterotomy combined with passage of a Dormia basket or a balloon is still considered as gold standard. However, it is invasive and afflicted with a significant complication risk for the patient; therefore it is not performed any more as a solely diagnostic investigation. The positive results of endosonography for the proof of choledocholithiasis are due to the good representability (in particular extrahepatic) of the biliary system. In contrast, the limited penetration depth of the hepatic hilus and the right bile duct parts may be evaluated conditionally. The results of the extraductal EUS with mini-probes for an exact determination of choledocholithiasis are promising[20].

PAPILLA

Endosonography is the only secure imaging technique for the diagnosis of pathological variances of the papilla, even if prospective multicentre studies are missing. Before ablation of a papillary adenoma EUS should be performed on the one hand to determine the depth of tumour infiltration and on the other hand to exclude a secondary tumour localized more proximally to the bile duct area.

PANCREAS

Chronic pancreatitis

EUS has a high diagnostic accuracy in the diagnosis and therapy planning of chronic pancreatitis, based on the high local resolution and the subsequent judgement clarity of parenchymal and ductal criteria[21].

> *Note 11*: Endoscopic ultrasound is a suitable method for the early diagnosis of chronic pancreatitis, for the clarification of stenosis of the pancreatic duct, and for decision-making in pseudocysts.

Despite differences in examination procedures and reduced concordance of distinct experienced examiners regarding the endosonographic diagnosis of chronic pancreatitis, the excellent diagnostic yield is valid both for radial and longitudinal EUS.

The original 13 criteria for the diagnosis of chronic pancreatitis suggested by Lees[22] were evaluated by Wiersema et al. in 1993[23] and later modified. Calcifications and/or concrements of the pancreatic duct were findings with a safe (100%) predictive value in 30 patients definitive with documented chronic pancreatitis. The demonstration of single parenchymal criteria with the exception of calcifications as early signs of a chronic pancreatitis may not be overestimated. The nine criteria from the study of Wiersema et al. (five ductal and four parenchymal criteria) underlie most published studies of EUS in chronic pancreatitis (Table 4).

Table 4 Endosonographic criteria of the pancreatic duct and parenchyma of chronic pancreatitis by Lees[22] 1986 and Wiersema et al. 1993[23]

Ductal criteria	Parenchymal criteria
Increased echogen contour of the pancreatic duct	Echogene reflexes (12 mm)
Irregular contour of the main pancreatic duct	Accented lobularity (2–5 echopoor zones surrounded by echogene septal cystic mass)
Dilated side branches (corpus/ cauda)	Focal hypoechoic zones
Concrements of the pancreatic duct	Parenchymal cysts (>2 mm)
Dilation of the main pancreatic duct (caput >3 mm, corpus >2 mm, cauda >1 mm)	Echogene irregular striped structures ('wisps')*
	Enlargement of the organ*
Constriction with dilation of the main duct *	
Abruption of duct with cystic formation*	

* Only in criteria list of Lees.

Note 12: Detection of 'calcifications' and/or 'pancreatic concrements' have the highest diagnostic impact for the diagnosis of chronic pancreatitis.

Anatomical variants of Pancreas divisum

Anatomical variants of the pancreatic duct can be diagnosed by endosonography. Characteristics of a pancreas divisum are a ventral pancreatic duct outgoing of the Papilla Vateri which cannot be further pursued from the ventral portion into the dorsal portion or cannot be identified in the ventral portion. Vice-versa, a pancreas divisum can be excluded if the pancreatic duct can be pursued in its course continuously between ventral and dorsal part and/or between the origin of the papilla vateri and the genu pancreatis (Y-sign).

For the diagnosis of chronic pancreatitis the sensitivity of endosonography is comparable to endoscopic retrograde cholangiopancreatography (ERCP) and may even replace it for solely diagnostic indications. Due to the high variability of normal findings, the specificity of EUS – just like ERCP and functional tests – definitively depends on the examined collectives and/or in individual cases on the clinical setting. Without appreciation of clinical data and the patients' history, chronic pancreatitis is frequently misdiagnosed. A definite statement on the presence of a chronic pancreatitis is impossible when investigations are performed shortly after acute pancreatitis (approximately 4 weeks).

DUCTAL ADENOCARCINOMA

EUS is the most sensitive technique for the detection of pancreatic masses apart from multidetector CT. It has an accuracy of 78–94% concerning T-staging and 64–82% concerning N-staging. In comparison of the different methods, a superiority of endosonography for tumour description was documented with a positive predictive value of 97% ($n = 237$). In contrast, ERCP led only in 92% ($n = 126$), angiography in 88% ($n = 42$), CT in 76% ($n = 180$) and transabdominal ultrasound in only 73% ($n = 210$) to the diagnosis of pancreatic carcinoma. In patients with smaller pancreatic tumours (<3 cm) the superiority of endosonography is even more obvious. EUS is the method of the choice for the exclusion of a pancreatic mass with unclear clinical or imaging findings. The highest advantages of the EUS are for tumours <3 cm (and still more clearly <2 cm).

Staging

Multidetector CT and the combination of transabdominal ultrasound and EUS represents nowadays the standard techniques for evaluation of primary tumour size and local tumour progression[24]. A comparison of the literature with respect to the preoperative staging of pancreatic carcinoma between EUS and CT resulted in summary in a slightly higher sensitivity for EUS. However, a high heterogeneity was demonstrated concerning design, quality and results, as well as clear methodical weaknesses with the comparison of the studies. A literature research for MRI showed a high sensitivity and specificity for detection of a biliary obstruction. However, a smaller sensitivity was demonstrated for differentiation between a benign and malignant obstruction.

Even if the peripancreatic lymph nodes can be identified with high sensitivity, it remains difficult to differentiate between infiltrated malignant lymph nodes and reactively modified lymph nodes.

The endosonographic proof of a vascular infiltration was recently published by Brugge et al. and other groups, and indicated an accuracy of 55–94%[25]. As a sign of vascular infiltration a loss of vascular wall layering between tumour and vessel lumen, an irregularly developed vascular wall, the detection of tumour within the vessel, as well as the detection of collaterals may be present. A clear demarcation of the intima almost certainly excludes an infiltration of the vessels. Most studies show substantial restrictions due to high interobserver variability. In recently published studies the results for EUS in evaluation of resectability were clearly worse. However, the sensitivity and specificity were postulated to be lower than 80% by the group of Rösch.

DIFFERENTIAL DIAGNOSIS OF PANCREATIC LESIONS

With proof of a definite pancreatic tumour and urgent suspicion of a ductal adenocarcinoma of the pancreas without distant metastasis and existing option of curative surgery, an operation is primarily indicated and no puncture to obtain histology is necessary.

However, this does not mean that each pancreatic mass should undergo surgery unreflected, but rather that the options of the preoperative (in particular the imaging) diagnostics must be exhausted. In disagreement with formerly published statements that 95% of all pancreatic tumours are ductal adenocarcinomas, it can be shown that in specialized centres up to 50% of these masses are other tumour entities. Thus, it is of crucial importance to clarify the dignity of such a mass preoperatively, since significant operation lethality has to be considered.

Thus, the quality of the preoperative diagnostics of an interdisciplinary centre can also be rated on the basis of preoperative correctly identified diagnoses, for example not leading to a modified Whipple Kausch operation. This in particular holds true for the asymptomatic serous microcystic pancreatic adenomas, which usually do not degenerate, and inflammatory pancreatic variances such as autoimmune pancreatitis, to be treated with corticosteroids. Differentiated neuroendocrine tumours should be enucleated (if possible), preserving pancreatic tissue (considering appropriate criteria, for example a tumour distance of >5 mm (–10) mm to the main pancreatic duct, etc.) and should not undergo radical operation techniques.

Note 14: The priority of endoscopic ultrasound can be summarized as follows: (a) exclusion of pancreatic tumours, (b) characterization of pancreatic tumours inclusive punctures with cytological investigation, (c) staging of malignant pancreatic tumours, (d) application in the context of neoadjuvant therapy concepts.

Cystic pancreatic lesions

At least four different types of cystic neoplasia are described in the literature and listed in the WHO classification (serous (micro-, oligo-, and macrocystic) adenoma (SCA), mucinous cystadenoma and cystadenocarcinoma (MCA), intraductal papillary mucinous neoplasia (IPMN), and pseudopapillary cystic neoplasia), which must be distinguished from pseudocysts. In a study on 341 patients cystic fluid was examined for CEA, CA 72-4, CA 125, CA 19-9, and CA 15-3. The definite histological diagnosis was confirmed in 112 patients by surgical resection (including 68 mucinous neoplasia, seven serous cystic neoplasia, 27 inflammatory pseudotumours as well as five endocrine tumours and five other entities).

A critical CEA value of 192 ng/ml could be determined by analysing the data, permitting at least the differentiation of mucinous versus non-mucinous cystic lesions with a sensitivity of 73% and a specificity of 84%. There were no combined parameters, showing better accuracy than the exclusive CEA determination.

Table 5 Indications for anal and rectal ultrasound examinations

Anal cancer	T and N staging
Rectal cancer	T and N staging
Tumour follow-up	Submucosal and extrarectal recurrences
Incontinence	Evaluation of sphincter morphology
Extrarectal pathologies	Abscesses, fistulas, liquid and solid masses
Interventions	Diagnostic and therapeutic punctures

ENDORECTAL ULTRASOUND

Endosonographic examinations (endorectal ultrasound; ERUS) of the perineum, anus and rectum including the surrounding structures have become increasingly important over recent years. While ERUS displays primarily the layers of the rectal wall and its environment, anal endosonography is used to evaluate the sphincter musculature and the pelvic base. The indications for anal and rectal ultrasound examinations are summarized in Table 5.

Staging

Since during therapy planning in neoadjuvant procedures the exact tumour stage cannot be defined by the pathological-anatomically surgical preparation, the meaning of EUS regarding the exact preoperative staging is still higher compared to definitive postoperative therapy strategies. This is in particular true for an exact differentiation of early stages (T1/T2) and locally advanced stages (T3/T4 +/–N). While the sensitivity and specificity of EUS show satisfactory security for the determination of the T stage in early stages of rectal carcinoma, the differentiation between T2 and T3 tumours, differing often only by small spiculae with an excess of the muscularis propria from each other, remain difficult.

In comparison to T-staging, the evaluation of lymph node status has a larger range for false diagnosis, since hypoechoic lymph node structures may be modified due to both inflammation and metastasis, whereby with increasing size of the lymph node the probability for malignant change clearly increases. In cases of doubt some authors recommend an endosonographically guided puncture (FNA, with linear echoscopes); however, a negative biopsy does not prove a N0 status.

ERUS is regarded as obligatory by the interdisciplinary guidelines of the German cancer society (Deutsche Krebsgesellschaft e.V.) if a local excision is planned in assumed T1 tumours with histomorphological signs of low-grade carcinoma. The results of ERUS regarding the T- and N-staging of primary rectal tumours are summarized in Tables 6 and 7 (studies with more than 100 patients).

Furthermore, in the tumour follow-up setting EUS is highly relevant and is recommended in the interdisciplinary guidelines 2000 as a follow-up

Table 6   T-staging of primary rectal tumours

Author	Year	n	Accuracy	Sensitivity	Specificity	PPV	NPV
Nielsen et al.	1996	100	94	96	87	96	87
Rifkin et al.	1989	101	72	67	77	73	72
Rafaelsen et al.	1994	107	89	96	77	88	91
Fedyaev et al.	1995	109	95	97	91	96	94
Glaser et al.	1990	110	94	96	91	92	96
Katsura et al.	1992	112	97	96	100	100	94
Herzog et al.	1993	118	93	98	75	90	95
Yamashita et al.	1988	122	86	96	52	88	78
Akasu et al.	1997	150	89	96	78	88	91
Sailer et al.	1997	162	89	97	81	83	97
Garcia-Aguilar et al.	2002	545	69	–	–	72	93

n, number; PPV, positive predictive value; NPV, negative predictive value.

Table 7   N-staging of primary rectal tumours

Author	Year	n	Accuracy	Sensitivity	Specificity	PPV	NPV
Rifkin et al.	1989	102	81	50	92	68	84
Fedyaev et al.	1995	109	72	94	55	61	92
Herzog et al.	1993	111	80	89	73	71	90
Hildebrandt et al.	1990	113	79	72	83	72	83
Akasu et al.	1997	164	76	77	74	79	72
Garcia-Aguilar et al.	2002	238	64	33	64	52	68

n, number; PPV, positive predictive value; NPV, negative predictive value.

examination, particularly in stage UICC II and III tumours[28]. The advantage of EUS is the detection of submucosal and pararectal (extrarectal) pathologies remaining inaccessible for rectal digital investigation and endoscopy due to their extraluminal localization. A further advantage is the ability to take targeted transmural biopsies. Recurrent disease presents typically as an echopoor mass, whereby it is clearly not possible to differentiate between a recurrence of a malignancy and any scar formation solely by the imaging technique.

ANAL ENDOSONOGRAPHY IN INCONTINENCE

An exact knowledge of the individual anatomical and functional defects of the sphincter apparatus and the surrounding structures is obligatory for choosing a rational therapy of anal incontinence considering the appropriate differential diagnostic and different aetiologies. Therefore, anal EUS is used as an important imaging technique and minimally invasive procedure in the clarification of faecal incontinence.

Currently four main forms of anal incontinence were described based on the combination of EUS and rectal perfusions-manometry, i.e. a purely sensory form, a predominantly muscular form, a combination of both as well as a disturbance of the reservoir function of the rectum, which may have different therapeutic options. Publications from the early 1990s underline the value of anal EUS, which could point out that a considerable number of patients, who had been formerly classified as 'idiopathic incontinence', actually showed sonomorphological sphincter damage. However, endosonographically detectable changes seem to be only clinically and/or functionally relevant, if accordingly correlations with clinical and/or functional parameters exist, e.g. manometry-determined sphincter pressures.

Fistula

Another important application of ERUS exists in the diagnostics and demarcation of anal fistula, in particular for complex fistulas, as for instance in recurrent or underlying Crohn's disease. The representation of the puborectal loop and muscularis levator ani is crucial. The distinction between pelvirectal (suprasphincteric) and ischiorectal (infrasphincteric) localization of abscesses and fistulas is possible with ERUS.

Endosonographically-guided interventions

Currently, only a few studies are available with respect to transrectal biopsy of non-urological and/or non-gynaecological tumours, although they are generally possible. Due to the outstanding resolution of ERUS it is suitable in particular for detection of small amounts of liquid in the small pelvis. Besides, for the exact relations of the lesion with neighbouring organs and/or structures ERUS may be performed before biopsy, so that a safe puncture of relevant liquid structures can usually be performed with a transrectal approach.

Colon (proximal to the rectum)

Endosonographic examination of the colon with conventional orthograd and also side-viewing echoendoscopes, and in addition with mini-probe technology, is possible, but this technique has so far not been established in the daily setting.

Mediastinum

Malignant mediastinal lymph nodes are observed for example in about 5% of patients with ductal pancreatic adenocarcinoma and exclude surgery[29]. Thus, evaluation of the mediastinal lymph node stations is essential to each gastroenterologist performing endosonographic examinations. However, the specific (pneumological) indications are beyond the scope of this review of endosonographic techniques.

Adrenal gland

Within the past 10 years, endosonographic detection of the adrenal glands was established. Kenneth Chang and co-workers published for the first time the definability of the left adrenal gland (97%) in 31 patients. The access and sonomorphology were described and validated simultaneously in 154 patients[30].

The indications for endosonographic adrenal gland diagnosis from a gastroenterological point of view can be summarized as follows:

1. Detection of metastasis of the adrenal gland.

2. Characterization of unclear CT and MRI findings, in particular small adrenal tumours by layer affiliation and analysis of tumour-typical characteristics in patients with gastrointestinal tumours.

3. Clarification of the dignity of adrenal gland tumours by puncture (FNA) if necessary.

Endosonographically guided transgastral puncture for differential diagnosis (metastasis versus incidentaloma) is possible, also in very small tumours, particularly on the left side, with a minimal risk of complications and excellent diagnostic results of the puncture. The cannula diameter should be chosen as small as possible, due to satisfactory cytology.

Portal hypertension

Numerous studies were performed in patients with portal hypertension; none of them could show any therapeutic or clinical relevance.

Therapeutic endosonography

Endosonography contributes substantially to both interdisciplinary planning and the therapy of pancreatic pseudocysts, peripancreatic necroses[31], pancreatic duct obstructions, bile duct stenosis, pancreatic concrements, and changes of the papilla. In addition, EUS-guided cholangiodrainage, rendezvous procedures and further more minimally invasive indications fascinate within the application of EUS. However, therapeutic EUS is beyond the scope of this chapter.

References

1. Fusaroli P, Vallar R, Togliani T, Khodadadian E, Caletti G. Scientific publications in endoscopic ultrasonography: a 20-year global survey of the literature. Endoscopy. 2002;34:451–6.
2. Lambert R, Caletti G, Cho E et al. International Workshop on the clinical impact of endoscopic ultrasound in gastroenterology. Endoscopy. 2000;32:549–84.
3. Dietrich CF, Ignee A, Frey H. Contrast-enhanced endoscopic ultrasound with low mechanical index: a new technique. Z Gastroenterol. 2005;43:1219–23.

4. Adler DG, Jacobson BC, Davila RE et al. ASGE guideline: complications of EUS. Gastrointest Endosc. 2005;61:8–12.

5. Jenssen C. Complications of endoscopic ultrasound in 18 German centers – report of a survey, 2004. Unpublished data.

6. Meining A, Dittler HJ, Wolf A et al. You get what you expect? A critical appraisal of imaging methodology in endosonographic cancer staging. Gut. 2002;50:599–603.

7. Pech O, May A, Gunter E, Gossner L, Ell C. The impact of endoscopic ultrasound and computed tomography on the TNM staging of early cancer in Barrett's esophagus. Am J Gastroenterol. 2006;101:2223–9.

8. May A, Gunter E, Roth F et al. Accuracy of staging in early oesophageal cancer using high resolution endoscopy and high resolution endosonography: a comparative, prospective, and blinded trial. Gut. 2004;53:634–40.

9. Gotoda T, Yanagisawa A, Sasako M et al. Incidence of lymph node metastasis from early gastric cancer: estimation with a large number of cases at two large centers. Gastric Cancer. 2000;3:219–25.

10. Radaszkiewicz T, Dragosics B, Bauer P. Gastrointestinal malignant lymphomas of the mucosa-associated lymphoid tissue: factors relevant to prognosis. Gastroenterology. 1992;102:1628–38.

11. Fischbach W, Goebeler-Kolve ME, Greiner A. Diagnostic accuracy of EUS in the local staging of primary gastric lymphoma: results of a prospective, multicenter study comparing EUS with histopathologic stage. Gastrointest Endosc. 2002;56:696–700.

12. Mallery S, Lai R, Bardales R, Stelow E, Debol S, Stanley M. EUS-guided needle aspiration (EUS-FNA) in subepithelial GI-tract masses (SIGIM): results in 105 lesions. Gastrointest Endosc. 2004;59:AB 234 (abstract).

13. Davila RE, Faigel DO. GI stromal tumors. Gastrointest Endosc. 2003;58:80–8.

14. Polkowski M, Butruk E. Submucosal lesions. Gastrointest Endosc Clin N Am. 2005;15:33–54, viii.

15. Gress F, Schmitt C, Savides T et al. Interobserver agreement for EUS in the evaluation and diagnosis of submucosal masses. Gastrointest Endosc. 2001;53:71–6.

16. Hizawa K, Kawasaki M, Kouzuki T, Suekane H, Matsumoto T, Fujishima M. Endosonographic classifications of gastrointestinal submucosal tumors. Dig Endosc. 2000;12:120–5.

17. Krinsky ML, Savides TJ, Behling CA. *Ex-vivo* correlation of endosonographic features with pathologic findings in gastric stromal tumors. Gastrointest Endosc. 2001;53:AB 170 (abstract).

18. Polkowski M, Butruk E. Submucosal lesions. Gastrointest Endosc Clin N Am. 2005;15:33–54, viii.

19. Palazzo L, Landi B, Cellier C, Cuillerier E, Roseau G, Barbier JP. Endosonographic features predictive of benign and malignant gastrointestinal stromal cell tumours. Gut. 2000;46:88–92.

20. Seifert H, Wehrmann T, Hilgers R, Gouder S, Braden B, Dietrich CF. Catheter probe extraductal EUS reliably detects distal common bile duct abnormalities. Gastrointest Endosc. 2004;60:61–7.

21. Jenssen C, Dietrich CF. [Endoscopic ultrasound in chronic pancreatitis.]. Z Gastroenterol. 2005;43:737–49.

22. Lees WR. Endoscopic ultrasonography of chronic pancreatitis and pancreatic pseudocysts. Scand J Gastroenterol Suppl. 1986;123:123–9.

23. Wiersema MJ, Hawes RH, Lehman GA, Kochman ML, Sherman S, Kopecky KK. Prospective evaluation of endoscopic ultrasonography and endoscopic retrograde cholangiopancreatography in patients with chronic abdominal pain of suspected pancreatic origin. Endoscopy. 1993;25:555–64.

24. Rosch T, Dittler HJ, Strobel K et al. Endoscopic ultrasound criteria for vascular invasion in the staging of cancer of the head of the pancreas: a blind reevaluation of videotapes. Gastrointest Endosc. 2000;52:469–77.

25. Gress FG, Hawes RH, Savides TJ et al. Role of EUS in the preoperative staging of pancreatic cancer: a large single-center experience. Gastrointest Endosc. 1999;50:786–91.

26. Micames C, Jowell PS, White R et al. Lower frequency of peritoneal carcinomatosis in patients with pancreatic cancer diagnosed by EUS-guided FNA vs. percutaneous FNA. Gastrointest Endosc. 2003;58:690–5.

27. Levy MJ, Smyrk TC, Reddy RP et al. Endoscopic ultrasound-guided trucut biopsy of the cyst wall for diagnosing cystic pancreatic tumors. Clin Gastroenterol Hepatol. 2005;3:974–9.
28. Sailer M, Bussen D, Fein M et al. Endoscopic ultrasound-guided transrectal biopsies of pelvic tumors. J Gastrointest Surg. 2002;6:342–6.
29. Snady H, Bruckner H, Siegel J, Cooperman A, Neff R, Kiefer L. Endoscopic ultrasonographic criteria of vascular invasion by potentially resectable pancreatic tumors. Gastrointest Endosc. 1994;40:326–33.
30. Dietrich CF, Wehrmann T, Hoffmann C, Herrmann G, Caspary WF, Seifert H. Detection of the adrenal glands by endoscopic or transabdominal ultrasound. Endoscopy. 1997;29:859–64.
31. Seifert H, Faust D, Schmitt T, Dietrich C, Caspary W, Wehrmann T. Transmural drainage of cystic peripancreatic lesions with a new large-channel echo endoscope. Endoscopy. 2001;33:1022–6.

7
Innovations in endoscopic ultrasound

P. VILMANN and V. SHARMA

INTRODUCTION

Endoscopic ultrasound (EUS) combines two modalities: endoscopic visualization and high-frequency ultrasound, thereby permitting precise delineation of the individual layers of the gastrointestinal tract as well as adjacent surrounding structures and organs. Ever since the introduction of endosonography in the early 1980s the method has undergone immense development, leading to an important method for clinical decision-making in a variety of indications in gastroenterology, pulmonal medicine and oncology[1–4]. This development, leading to what EUS is today, are mainly due to innovations that are developed during different time periods and may as such be regarded in different phases.

The aim of this chapter is to highlight innovations important to the present status of EUS and to look into future perspectives of EUS imaging and interventions.

HISTORY OF EUS INNOVATIONS

The innovations of EUS can be regarded in three important steps, i.e. first development of EUS imaging with radial mechanical transducers, secondly, development of linear electronic transducer technology and finally development of EUS-guided intervention, including biopsy and therapeutic procedures (Table 1).

From 1980 to 1986 developments of endoscopes and miniprobes with mechanical transducers was initiated mainly by the Olympus company. Based on these developments numerous basic studies with delineation of the wall layers both under normal as well as abnormal conditions were published, and graduately indications for endosonography were established (Figure 1)[5,6].

During the period 1986–1991 the indications of EUS imaging with mechanical radial scanning transducers were established, including staging and evaluation of resectability of gastrointestinal (GI) cancer and GI lymphoma, evaluation of GI tract pathology (large gastric folds, submucosal tumours, impressions, vascular malformations etc.), evaluation of extrahepatic

Table 1 Important phases of EUS and its innovations

Time period	Innovations
1980–1986	Development of endoscopes and mini-probes with mechanical transducers and basic studies on EUS
1986–1991	Establishing indications of EUS imaging with mechanical transducers
1991–2000	Development of electronic transducer technology and beginning of EUS-FNA
2000–2008	Establishing indications of EUS-guided interventions (biopsy and therapy)

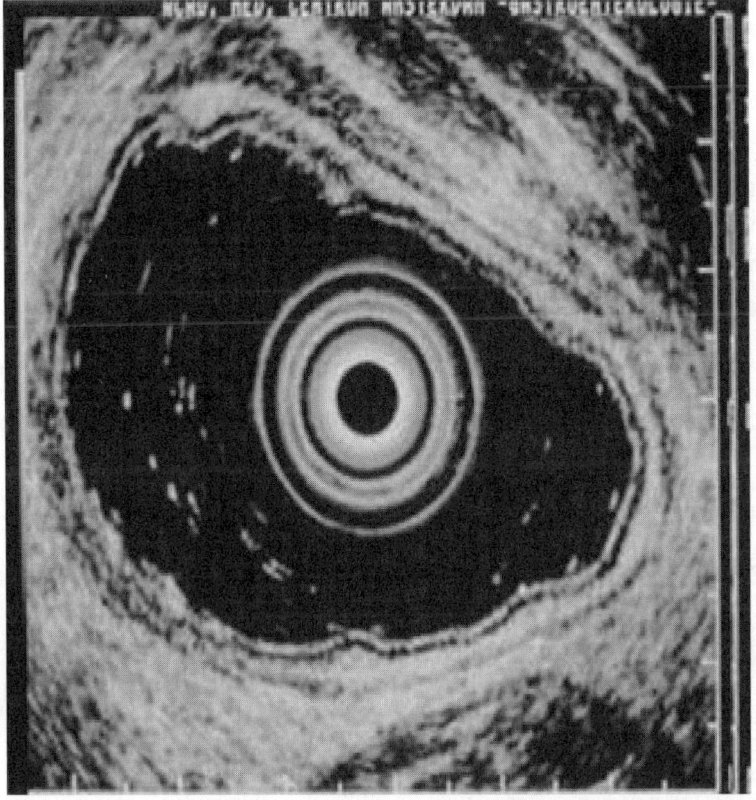

Figure 1 Radial mechanical EUS image demonstrating the normal gastric wall layers. Image courtesy of Dr Lok Tio (1986)

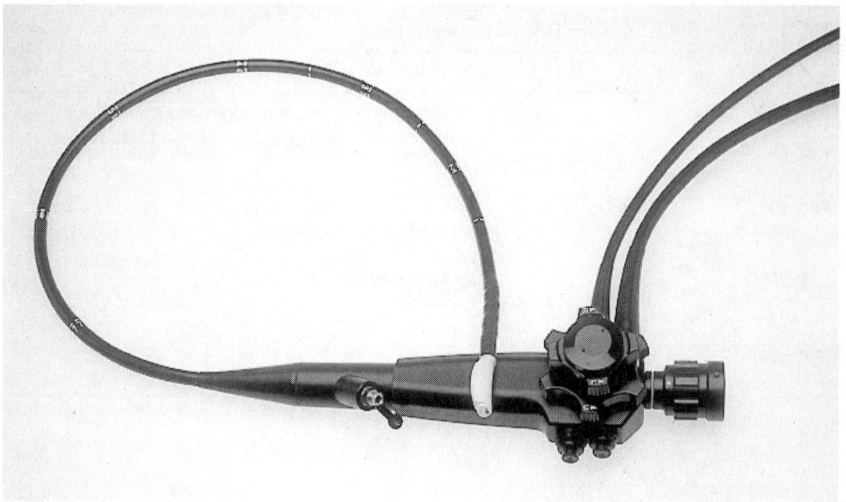

Figure 2   First prototype curved linear echoendoscope first used by the author in 1988 (Hitachi/ Pentax (EC 124))

obstruction, diagnosis of common bile duct stones and microlithiasis, evaluation of pancreatitis, detection of neuroendocrine tumours and evaluation of cystic pancreatic tumours[2–8].

The next important step was development of an endoscope with a curved linear electronic transducer. The first prototype that was really considered of value for human use was developed in 1988 by Hitachi/Pentax (EC 124) and first used by our group[9] (Figure 2). However, it soon became clear that a biopsy channel was needed.

Based on these experiences another echo-endoscope with a 2 mm biopsy channel was developed (Pentax/Hitachi, FG 32 UA) (Figure 3). This endoscope was used by our group in 1991.

From 1991 to 2000 further development of electronic transducer technology and EUS-FNA (fine needle aspiration) was done. Early needles testing for EUS-FNA was started by our group in 1991 in collaboration with Wilson Cook Denmark and the first EUS-guided FNA biopsy of a pancreatic lesion was performed in the same year (Figure 4)[10]. The first dedicated handle device with needle was created by our group during the period between 1991 and 1993 (Hancke/Vilmann needle, GIP/Medi-Globe, Achenmühle, Germany) (Figure 5)[11]. Gradually a variety of FNA needles with different diameters were developed by different companies from 1995 to 2000. All these devices were basicly similar to the original needle design.

Based on experiences from the late 1990s we realized the great potential of EUS-guided intervention. It became more and more clear that it was possible to reach regions in the human body that can either not be reached by other imaging modalities or are too minute to targeted trancutaneously.

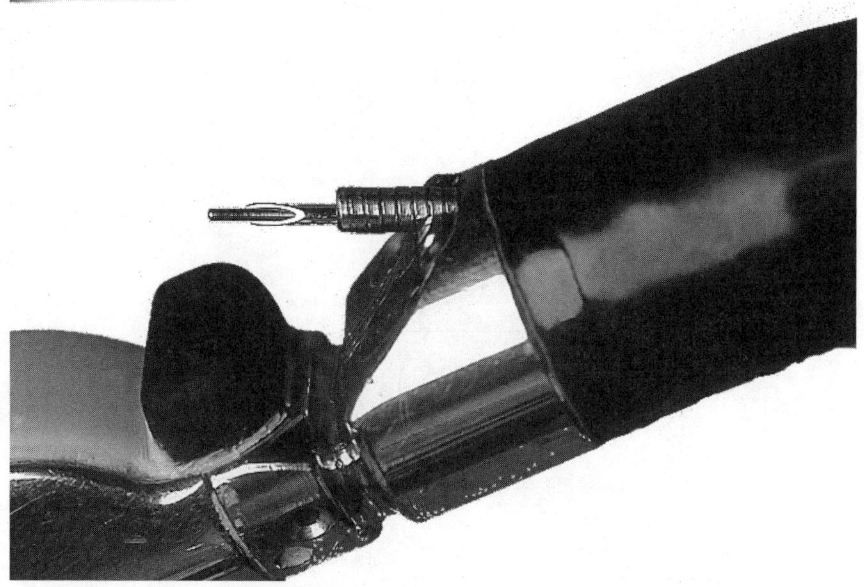

Figure 3 The first echo-endoscope with a 2 mm biopsy channel was developed by Pentax and Hitachi (FG 32 UA). The image shows part of the distal end and a needle extending from the biopsy channel outlet

During the years 2000–2008 the indications of EUS-guided interventions (biopsy and therapy) were developed and are now becoming routine practice.

The indications of EUS-FNA that are firmly established at present are EUS-guided biopsy of lesions for staging of gastrointestinal cancer and lung cancer, as well as primary diagnosis of mediastinal lesions, lymph nodes, gastrointestinal submucosal tumours, pancreatic and biliary tract pathologies, as well as adrenal gland masses[12–27].

Development of EUS-guided therapy may be regarded as a logical further step in EUS-guided intervention. At present a wide range of established indications for EUS-guided therapy, as well as many potential future applications, have been published. Some of these procedures are established clinically relevant procedures in humans, others are animal studies or phase I or II studies in humans. The therapeutic EUS procedures include injection and drainage procedures, and additional other procedures are in the pipeline, such as EUS-guided implantation, coagulation (radiofrequency and photodynamic therapy), resection of lesions and suturing. It may even be that EUS will gain an important role in natural orifice transluminal endoscopic surgery (NOTES).

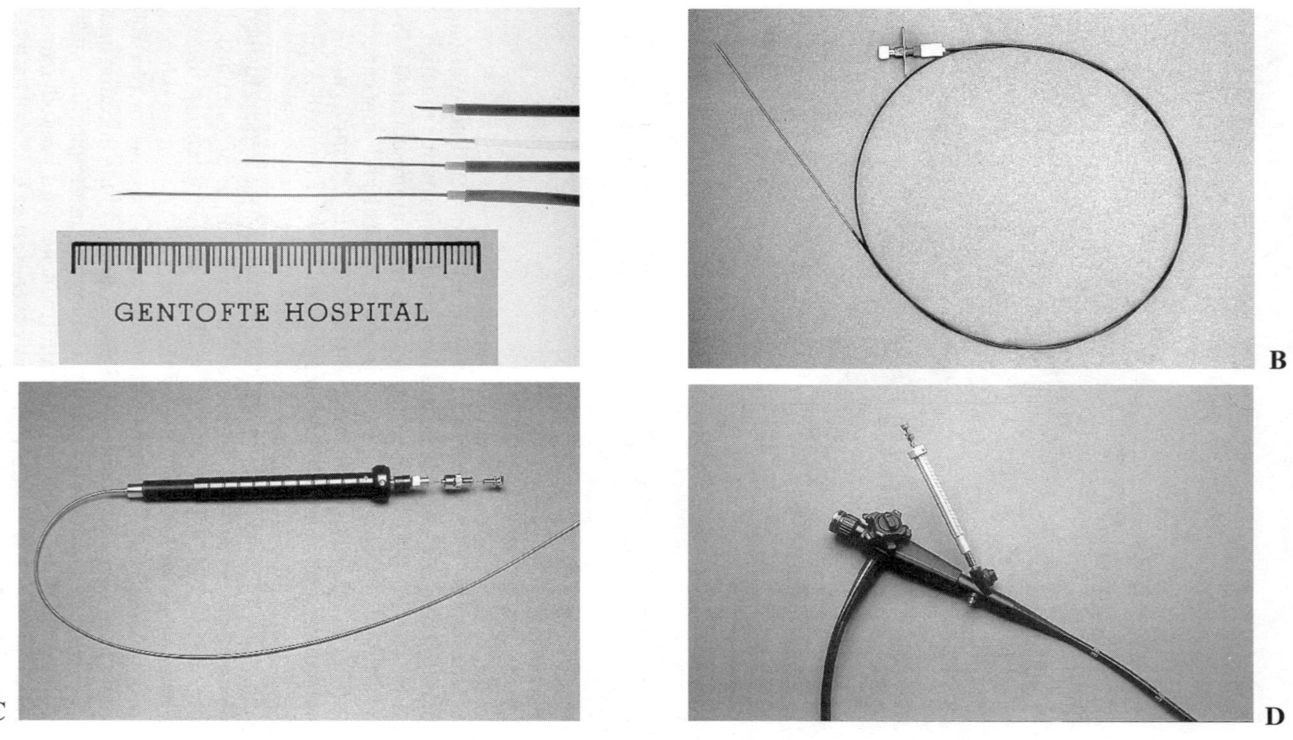

Figure 4 Early needles testing for EUS-FNA was started by our group in 1991 in collaboration with Wilson Cook Denmark, but shortly after taken over by GIP-Medizintechnik GmbH, Grassau). **A**: Different needle designs tested in the early phase of development of EUS-FNA. **B**: A long steel needle with a Teflon sheath (Wilson Cook, Denmark 1991). **C**: Prototype handle design for EUS-FNA composed of handle, needle piston, and sheath. **D**: Dedicated biopsy needle device luer-locked to the channel inlet of an EUS endoscope

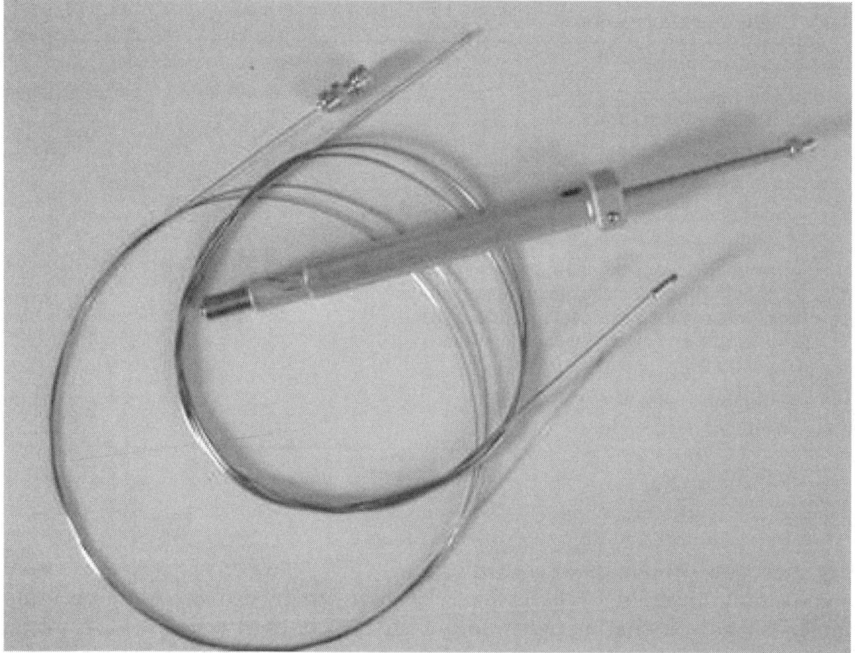

Figure 5 The first dedicated biopsy instrument for EUS-guided fine-needle biopsy was developed by one of the authors (P.V.) and Dr Søren Hancke in Denmark (GIP-Medizintechnik/ Medi-Globe GmbH, 1993). The device has three main interlocking components. The handle assembly is composed of handle, needle piston, and sheath

EUS-GUIDED INJECTION

Since the first description of EUS-FNA[10], the idea of EUS-guided injection in order to deliver substances into structures or lesions outlined by EUS has been an obvious challenge. The early reports of EUS-guided injections were injection of contrast media into dilated duct systems under fluoroscopy. EUS-guided injection has been utilized for cholangiography, lymphangiography and pancreatography with or without rendezvous-guidewire technique[28-35].

Since then a large number of case series and case reports have been published on different injection methods (Table 2)

COELIAC PLEXUS NEUROLYSIS

Pancreatic cancer and chronic pancreatitis produce chronic pain difficult to control. Coeliac plexus neurolysis (CPN) or block may provide significant relief. Wiersema and Wiersema[36] published a study of 58 patients undergoing EUS-CPN for inoperable pancreatic cancer pain. Pain scores were assessed using a standardized 11-point visual analogue scale. Forty-five patients (78%)

Table 2   EUS-guided injection

Coeliac plexus neurolysis

Injection in vascular lesions of the GI tract (Dieulafoy lesion, duodenal ulcer, gastrointestinal stromal tumour and varices)

Botulinum injection in achalasia

Injection in refractory oesophageal strictures

EUS-guided pancreatic cyst ablation

Anti-tumour therapy
    Ethanol lavage of pancreatic cystic neoplasms
    EUS-guided neuroendocrine tumour ablation
    Local chemotherapy of pancreatic neoplasms
    Immunotherapy of pancreatic neoplasms
    Gene therapy of pancreatic neoplasms

Cholangio, lymph-, and pancreatography

Tattooing of pancreatic lesions

---

experienced a drop in pain score after EUS-CPN. The overall pain scores were significantly lower ($p < 0.0001$) 2 weeks after the procedure. A multivariate analysis showed that patients found sustained pain relief for 24 weeks independent of morphine use or adjuvant therapy. However, patients who received chemotherapy alone or chemotherapy plus radiation had additional benefit.

Minor complications were postural hypotension (20%), diarrhoea (17%), and pain exacerbation (9%). At this time it is reasonable to conclude that EUS-CPN, when performed by experienced endosonographers, is a safe and efficient procedure, but additional studies are needed.

BOTULINUM INJECTION IN ACHALASIA

The thickened lower oesophageal sphincter (LOS) can be accurately visualized by EUS as an echo-poor structure in the lower oesophageal wall in patients with achalasia[37–43]. A few studies have described the use of EUS-directed injection of botulinum toxin selectively into the LOS in patients with achalasia[37,38,42]. However, no large randomized and controlled series comparing the blind endoscopic method with the EUS-guided method have been reported.

INJECTION THERAPY OF VASCULAR LESIONS

Catalano and colleagues[44] compared EUS-assisted sclerotherapy with band ligation of oesophageal varices; in a study of 14 patients, EUS-assisted sclerotherapy required significantly fewer sessions to achieve variceal obliteration, and it decreased the rate of rebleeding and mortality from recurrent variceal bleeding. Lahoti et al.[45] performed real-time EUS-guided sclerotherapy in five patients with non-bleeding oesophageal varices. There were no complications, and varices were obliterated in 2.2 sessions. They concluded that the confirmation of obliteration of varices, coupled with the ability to obliterate the perforating veins, which is not possible with standard sclerotherapy or banding techniques, might decrease the number of sessions and variceal recurrence.

Lee et al.[46] reported that bi-weekly EUS of gastric varices followed by injection of cyanoacrylate until gastric varix obliteration documentation by the absence of anechoic vascular structures in the gastric wall is effective. They found a statistically significant reduction ($p = 0.0053$) in the rebleeding rate compared with their non-EUS control group ($n = 47$). Michael J. Levy and colleagues recently published their experience regarding EUS-guided angiotherapy of refractory gastrointestinal bleeding[47].

STEROID INJECTION IN REFRACTORY GI TRACT STRICTURES

Endoscopic ultrasound miniprobe-assisted steroid injection in patients with refractory oesophageal strictures has been reported recently in a preliminary study in three patients[48]. After dilation of the stricture, 0.5 ml aliquots of steroid solution were injected in each of four quadrants at the thickest site of the stricture as judged by endosonography. All three patients had symptomatic improvement, but no long-term results are yet available.

ANTICANCER THERAPY

EUS has focused attention on the large group of upper GI malignancy patients who either have disseminated disease or in whom therapeutic options are limited due to concurrent disease. The search for more effective treatment strategies, including new methods for directed tumour destruction, have intensified, and following the introduction of EUS-FNA, EUS-directed tumour therapy seems to be, at least in theory, a new option for more intensive and accurate targeted therapy. EUS-directed tumour therapy can be applied to the primary tumour (e.g. liver, pancreas, stomach), to malignant lymph nodes, or to metastases within the liver parenchyma.

Chang et al.[49] published their preliminary data from a phase I clinical trial using EUS-directed immunotherapy. They examined the feasibility and safety of direct injection of cytoimplant under EUS guidance in eight patients with unresectable pancreatic adenocarcinoma, The median survival was 13.2 months. Major complications including bone marrow toxicity, haemorrhagic, infectious, renal, or cardiopulmonary toxicity were absent. This study showed that local immunotherapy is feasible and safe.

The technique of EUS-guided fine-needle injection (EUS-FNI) was recently applied to deliver antitumour viral therapy[50]. ONYX-015 (dll520) is an EIB-55-kDa gene-deleted replication-selective adenovirus that preferentially replicates in and kills malignant cells. Twenty-one patients with locally advanced adenocarcinoma of the pancreas or with metastatic disease, but minimal or absent liver metastases, underwent eight sessions of ONYX-015 delivered by EUS injection into the primary pancreatic tumour over 8 weeks. The final four treatments were given in combination with gemcitabine (intravenously, 1000 mg/m^2). After combination therapy, two patients had partial regressions of the injected tumour, two had minor responses, six had stable disease, and 11 had progressive disease.

The most recent EUS-guided antitumour therapy involves a novel gene therapy. TNFerade is a replication-deficient adeno-vector containing human tumour necrosis factor alpha (TNF-α) gene, regulated by a radiation-inducible promoter Egr-1[51]. The study design consisted of a 5-week treatment of weekly intratumoral injections of TNFerade. EUS-guided FNI was compared with percutaneous approaches (computed tomography or ultrasound). TNFerade was combined with continuous intravenous 5-fluorouracyl (5-FU) and radiation. Four patients underwent resection, and one of these patients had a complete pathological response.

PANCREATIC CYST ABLATION

High-resolution ultrasound imaging provides a detailed evaluation and directs FNA in pancreatic cystic neoplastic lesions. EUS-guided ethanol lavage may offer an alternative to surgical resection of cystic neoplasm. Only thin-walled lesions with a diameter between 1 and 5 cm and unilocular lesions are ideal. In the first step of lavage the cyst is aspirated with a 22 gauge needle. The cyst fluid is evacuated until the cyst collapses. With the needle in place, 80% ethanol is repeatedly injected and lavaged over a 5-min period[52]. The most common complication is transient abdominal pain in less than 10% of patients. Rarely patients have experienced transient pancreatitis.

In a recent study[53], 25 patients with pancreatic cystic lesions of unknown subtype underwent FNA and subsequent injection of variable concentrations of ethanol (0–95%). Twenty-three of the 25 patients had complete follow-up, by way of resection (five patients) or repeat imaging. Eight of the 23 patients had complete radiologic resolution. Five patients underwent subsequent resection and showed variable degrees of epithelial ablation. Long-term studies will be required to determine whether ethanol lavage is capable of preventing the development of malignancy.

NEUROENDOCRINE TUMOUR ABLATION

Surgical resection is currently considered the standard treatment of insulinomas. EUS-guided ethanol ablation of endocrine tumours was recently reported[54] in a 78-year-old female with poor general condition, and refusal of surgical resection. Total 8 ml, 95% ethanol was injected into the tumour. The patient exhibited no further hypoglycaemic episodes, and her general condition improved rapidly.

EUS-GUIDED DRAINAGE PROCEDURES

A growing number of EUS-guided drainage procedures have been reported parallel to the introduction of EUS endoscopes with working channels large enough to allow introduction of catheters and stents. These procedures may be entirely monitored on EUS but many of these require both monitoring by EUS and endoscopic visualization, either with the EUS endoscope itself or after exchange with a second endoscope. A variety of procedures have been described (Table 3), including pancreatic pseudocyst drainage, bile duct drainage, pancreatic duct drainage, abscess drainage, drainage of fluids, necrosectomy of pancreatic collection, gallbladder fossa fluid drainage, haematoma drainage, and percutaneous endoscopic US-guided gastrostomy[55–82].

Table 3 EUS-guided drainage procedures

Pseudocyst drainage
Abscess drainage
Necrosectomy
Gallbladder fossa fluid drainage
Haematoma drainage
Transmural cholecystostomy
Cholangio- or pancreatico-enterostomy
Hepaticogastrostomy or duodenostomy

Pseudocyst drainage

Endoscopic pseudocyst drainage by the transgastric and transduodenal route has some limitations due to the potential risk of puncture of vessels interposed between the cyst and the gastric wall, with the risk of haemorrhage. The risk of perforation is also high when endoscopically visible intraluminal bulging is absent[55,56]. EUS allows precise assessment of the cyst anatomy, including its location, possible feeding duct, and content, as well as the shortest path between the gastric or duodenal wall and the cyst. Thus the most optimal puncture site can be selected and puncture of interposed vessels avoided[57–67].

Despite the large amount of published literature, there are no randomized or controlled studies comparing different methods at present. Giovannini et al.[68] drained 35 pancreatic cysts under EUS guidance, 15 had pseudocysts and 20 had pancreatic abscesses. No major complications occurred. Seifert at al.[69] evaluated a new one-step stenting device using a large channel echoendoscope (3.2 mm) for pseudocyst drainage in six patients.

Binmoeller et al.[58] reported EUS-guided pseudocyst drainage in 27 patients with a mean cyst diameter of 11 cm. Pseudocyst puncture and drainage was successful in 25 patients and failed in two patients due to bleeding. Cyst infection occurred in 13 patients due to stent clogging. The success rate for endosonography-guided pseudocyst drainage was 78%.

Abscess drainage and necrosectomy

Abscess drainage and pancreatic necrosectomy have been described in a number of publications. The route of endoscopic entrance has been either via the upper or the lower GI tract. The locations of the abscesses have been variable, in mediastinum, upper and lower abdomen[68,70–74].

Transmural cholecystostomy

EUS-guided transmural cholecystostomy has been described by Lee et al.[76] Nine elderly or high-risk patients diagnosed with acute cholecystitis were included in the study. All inflamed gallbladders were drained, and most of these patients had clinical resolution of acute cholecystitis.

Cholangio-enterostomy

Trans-duodenal drainage, trans-gastric drainage and trans-jejunal drainage have been tried in patients in whom ERCP failed to drain the obstructed bile duct, or in patients with gastric outlet obstruction due to pyloric stenosis/ duodenal stenosis and/or Billroth II gastrectomy with Roux-en-Y anastomosis. Hepaticogastrostomy and choledochoduodenostomy have been described by various groups over the past 10 years[77–82]. The procedures may either be performed directed by EUS or partly directed and assisted by EUS. Several approaches have been described either via the duodenum or the stomach into the common bile duct, hepatic duct or intrahepatic duct system. Colour Doppler is used to identify the regional vasculature. Bile duct puncture with a 19 gauge needle is then performed under fluoroscopic and endosonographic control. After successful biliary access, bile is aspirated and contrast is injected under fluoroscopy to demonstrate biliary opacification. A guidewire is introduced through the EUS needle and advanced in an antegrade fashion, to cross the biliary obstruction and advance the guidewire into the duodenum. In cases in which the guidewire cannot be advanced across the obstruction, a transenteric fistula is created in an attempt to decompress the biliary tree. Stent insertion may be performed via the echoendoscope, by exchange of endoscopes or as a rendezvous procedure with ERCP.

Hepaticogastrostomy

This method was first described in 2003 by Giovannini and co-workers[77]. Burmester and co-workers[78] performed EUS-guided cholangio-drainage (ECD) in four cases, with successful 8.5 French stent placement in three and one bile leak as a complication. In two cases Mallery and co-workers[79] performed ECD by cannulation adjacent to a EUS-placed wire, with a minor complication of wire passage outside the bile duct lumen. Puspok and co-workers[80] reported a total of six successful ECD with no immediate complications. One bile leak was reported by Ponnudurai and co-workers[81] in a case of malignant biliary obstruction treated with EUS-guided hepaticogastrostomy and metal stenting. Kahaleh et al.[82] performed ECD in

23 patients; 17 had malignant strictures whereas six suffered benign conditions. Intrahepatic cholangiography was performed in 18 of the patients with conversion to an extrahepatic intervention in five (27%). Of the 13 patients undergoing intrahepatic intervention, 12 had a stent placed across the major papilla; a success rate of 92% was achieved in these patients. The individual with unsuccessful intervention suffered from primary sclerosing cholangitis with tortuous ducts and multiple strictures. The overall reported success rate of ECD was 89%, while an overall rate of complication was 18%, including three major complications. Other authors have also reported similar experiences.

MISCELLANEOUS EUS-GUIDED PROCEDURES

Various other therapeutic and diagnostic EUS-guided procedures are under development such as EUS-guided photodynamic therapy and radiofrequency ablation, implantation of fiducials and radioactive seeds, portal vein catheterization, TIPS (transluminal intrahepatic portosystemic shunt) via the stomach and hepatic veins and suturing for gastropexy and trans-gastric endosurgery

Photodynamic therapy and radiofrequency ablation

Chan and colleagues[83] conducted a study on feasibility and safety of EUS-guided photodynamic therapy of the pancreas in a porcine model after injection of porfimer sodium. A 19-gauge needle was inserted into the pancreas, the liver, the spleen, and the kidney under EUS guidance. A quartz optical fibre passed through the EUS needle for the procedure. Localized tissue necrosis was achieved in all organs, without significant complications.

EUS-guided radiofrequency ablation has been described by Carrara et al.[84] in 14 pigs, with 14 successful ablations of pancreatic tissue with a new flexible bipolar probe.

Implantation of fiducials

Pishvarian et al.[85] published their experience with EUS-guided fiducial placement for cyberknife radiotherapy of mediastinal and abdominal malignancies in 2006. Image-guided stereotactic radiosurgery was performed after radiographic markers (fiducials) implantation at the tumour site, which were later used as reference points by the system to target the radiation beams. EUS-guided fiducial placement was successful in a total of 11 of 13 patients (84.6%). A total of three to six fiducials were placed in each patient. The locations of the tumours were retrocrural area, porta hepatis, gastro-oesophageal junction, mediastinum, thoracic paraspinal area, and pancreas.

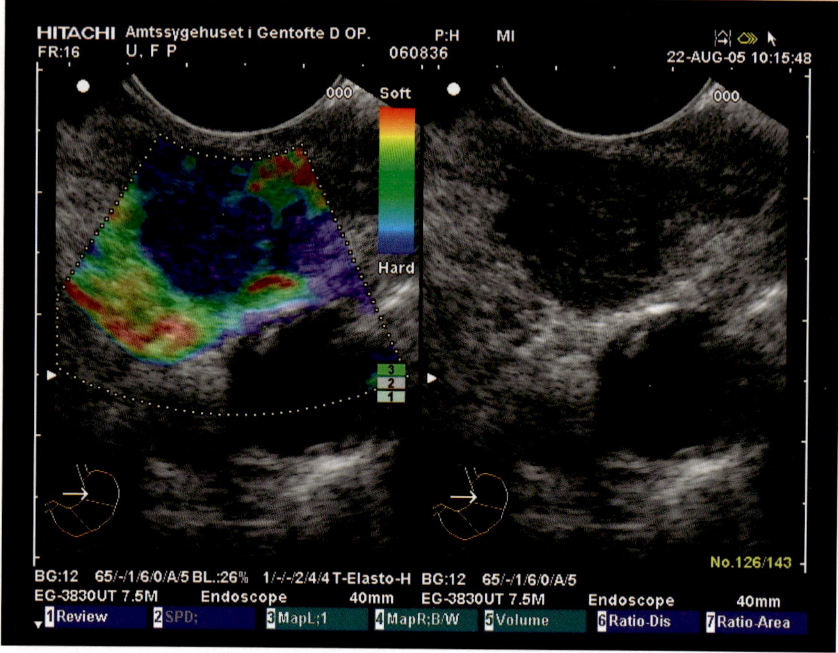

Figure 6 Tactile imaging: the image demonstrates a frozen still image of a malignant lesion obtained during real-time EUS elastography. The lesion is mainly displayed in blue demonstrating that this lesion is harder than its surroundings

Brachytherapy

Jin and colleagues[86] published a prospective pilot study in 2008, with endoscopic ultrasonography-guided interstitial implantation of iodine-125 seeds combined with chemotherapy for the treatment of unresectable pancreatic carcinoma. A total of 22 patients were included and all had successful implantation of iodine-125 seeds guided by EUS, with a median of 10 seeds and a maximum of 30 seeds per procedure.

In another pilot study published by Sun and colleagues[87] in 2006, EUS-guided interstitial brachytherapy of unresectable pancreatic cancer was performed in 15 patients. A mean number of 22 radioactive seeds per patient were implanted. There was moderate local tumour effect and follow-up showed some clinical benefit in 30% of the patients in this study.

Natural orifice transluminal endoscopic surgery (NOTES)

Fritscher-Ravens et al.[88–91] have published their experience with new trans-gastric endosurgical approaches to lymph nodes including node tagging, guidewire-directed hot biopsy, suturing, trans-gastric lymphadenectomy, trans-gastric gastropexy and hiatal hernia repair for gastro-oesophageal reflux disease under EUS control in a porcine model. These procedures seem to underline the potential of future developments in EUS-guided surgery.

FUTURE DEVELOPMENTS IN EUS

Innovations in EUS have mainly been driven from improvements in imaging, and with the development of linear electronic transducer technology, EUS-guided interventions. Improvement in electronic transducer technology and image software are rapidly being launched, and already being tested, such as three-dimensional imaging, tissue harmonic imaging, second harmonic imaging, pulse inversion, and power pulse inversion[92–95].

Tactile imaging during EUS procedures is currently under development by different companies, and several studies are already published[94,95] (Figure 6). The principle of real-time ultrasound elastography is based on initial tissue compression which produces strain (deformation) within the tissue, while the strain is smaller in harder tissue as compared to softer tissue. Consequently, by measuring the tissue strain induced by compression, it is possible to estimate the tissue mechanical properties, which may be useful in diagnosing and differentiating malignant tumours. The distribution of tissue elasticity is calculated in real time, and the result of the examination is displayed on the screen as a transparent overlay colour-coded image, together with the conventional grey-scale image of the examined structure.

Potential future indications of elastography are: selection of lymph nodes for EUS-FNA if they are multiple, exclusion of EUS-FNA in selected cases, evaluation of focal lesions of the pancreas, targeted biopsy (lymph nodes, pancreatic masses), evaluation of submucosal tumours, adrenal masses and acute pancreatitis.

Improvements in echo contrasts may lead not only to better differentiation of lesions, but also to possible targeted drug delivery. Image fusion between EUS and magnetic resonance or compound tomography seems to be promising and has already been shown to simplify EUS orientation[96].

There is a huge need for improvements in accessories for EUS-guided interventions such as better stents for drainage, better needle designs including histological needles, radiofrequency probes, cryoterm probes, etc.

It is expected that future developments in EUS imaging, as well as EUS-guided interventions, will increase the importance of EUS in the management of a variety of disorders in the human body. The combination of high-resolution imaging and precise targeting of minute lesions makes EUS a true minimally invasive modality.

References

1. Nickl NJ, Bhutani MS, Catalano MF et al. Clinical implications of endoscopic ultrasound: the American Endosonography Club Study. Gastrointest Endosc. 1996;44:371–7.
2. Tio TL, Tytgat GN. Endoscopic ultrasonography of normal and pathologic upper gastrointestinal wall structure. Comparison of studies *in vivo* and *in vitro* with histology. Scand J Gastroenterol Suppl. 1986;123:27–33.

3. Tio TL, Tytgat GN. Endoscopic ultrasonography in analysing peri-intestinal lymph node abnormality. Preliminary results of studies *in vitro* and *in vivo*. Scand J Gastroenterol Suppl. 1986;123:158–63.

4. Tio TL, Tytgat GN. Endoscopic ultrasonography in staging local resectability of pancreatic and periampullary malignancy. Scand J Gastroenterol Suppl. 1986;123:135–42.

5. Kimmey MB, Martin RW, Haggitt RC, Wang KY, Franklin DW, Silverstein FE. Histologic correlates of gastrointestinal ultrasound images. Gastroenterology. 1989;96:433–41.

6. Yasuda K, Tanaka Y, Fujimoto S, Nakajima M, Kawai K. Use of endoscopic ultrasonography in small pancreatic cancer. Scand J Gastroenterol Suppl. 1984;102:9–17.

7. Vilmann P et al. Guidelines of the European Society of Gastrointestinal Endoscopy (ESGE). Endoscopic Ultrasonography. Part I: Technique and upper GI tract. In cooperation with the European Endosonography Club Working Party. Endoscopy. 1996;28:474–9.

8. Vilmann P et al. Guidelines of the European Society of Gastrointestinal Endoscopy (ESGE). Endoscopic Ultrasonography. Part II: Retroperitoneum and Large Bowel, Training. In cooperation with the European Endosonography Club Working Party. Endoscopy. 1996;28:626–8.

9. Vilmann P, Hancke S, Khattar S. Endoscopic ultraonography of the upper gastrointestinal tract using a curved array transducer. A preliminary report. Surg Endosc. 1991;5:79–82.

10. Vilmann P, Jacobsen GK, Henriksen FW. Endoscopic ultrasonography with guided fine needle aspiration biopsy in pancreatic disease. A new diagnostic procedure. Gastrointest Endosc. 1992;38:172–3.

11. Vilmann P, Hancke S. A new biopsy handle instrument for endoscopic ultrasound guided biopsy. Gastrointest Endosc. 1996;43:238–42.

12. Vilmann P, Krasnik M, Larsen SS, Jacobsen GK, Clementsen P. Endoscopic trans-esophageal and endoscopic trans-bronchial ultrasound guided biopsy: a combined approach in the evaluation of mediastinal lesions. Endoscopy. 2005;37:833–9.

13. Antillon MR, Chang KJ. Endoscopic and endosonography guided fine-needle aspiration. Gastrointest Endosc Clin N Am. 2000;10:619–36.

14. Mertz H, Gautam S. The learning curve for EUS-guided FNA of pancreatic cancer. Gastrointest Endosc. 2004;59:33–7.

15. Wiersema MJ, Vilmann P, Giovannini M et al. Endosonography-guided fine-needle aspiration biopsy: diagnostic accuracy and complication assessment. Gastroenterology. 1997;112:1087–95.

16. Gress F, Gottlieb K, Sherman S et al. Endoscopic ultrasonography-guided fine-needle aspiration biopsy of suspected pancreatic cancer. Ann Intern Med. 2001;20:459–64.

17. Wallace MB, Kennedy T, Durkalski V et al. Randomized controlled trial of EUS-guided fine needle aspiration techniques for the detection of malignant lymphadenopathy. Gastrointest Endosc. 2001;54:441–7.

18. Fritscher-Ravens A, Bohuslavizki KH, Brandt L et al. Mediastinal lymph node involvement in potentially resectable lung cancer: comparison of CT, positron emission tomography, and endoscopic ultrasonography with and without fine-needle aspiration. Chest. 2003;123:442–519.

19. Nguyen P, Feng JC, Chang KJ et al, Endoscopic ultrasound (EUS) and EUS-guided fine-needle aspiration (FNA) of liver lesions. Gastrointest Endosc. 1999;50:357–61.

20. Ten Berge J, Hoffman BJ, Hawes RH et al. EUS-guided fine needle aspiration of the liver: indications, yield, and safety based on an international survey of 167 cases. Gastrointest Endosc. 2002;55:859–62.

21. Awad SS, Fagan S, Abudayyeh S et al. Preoperative evaluation of hepatic lesions for the staging of hepatocellular and metastatic liver carcinoma using endoscopic ultrasonography. Am J Surg. 2002;184:601–4.

22. Matsui M, Goto H, Niwa Y et al. Preliminary results of fine needle aspiration biopsy histology in upper gastrointestinal submucosal tumors. Endoscopy. 1998;30:750–5.

23. Ando N, Goto H, Niwa Y et al. The diagnosis of GI stromal tumors with EUS-guided fine needle aspiration with immunohistochemical analysis. Gastrointest Endosc. 2002;55:37–43.

24. Itoi T, Takei K, Sofuni A et al. Immunohistochemical analysis of p53 and MIB-1 in tissue specimens obtained from endoscopic ultrasonography-guided fine-needle aspiration biopsy for the diagnosis of solid pancreatic masses. Oncol Rep. 2005;13:229–34.

25. Ribeiro A, Vazquez-Sequeiros E, Wiersema LM et al. EUS-guided fine-needle aspiration combined with flow-cytometry and immunocytochemistry in the diagnosis of lymphoma. Gastrointest Endosc. 2001;53:485–91.

26. Takahashi K, Yamao K, Okubo K et al. Differential diagnosis of pancreatic cancer and focal chronic pancreatitis by using EUS-guided FNA. Gastrointest Endosc. 2005;61:76–9.

27. Jacobson BC, Pitman MB, Brugge WR et al. EUS-guided fine needle aspiration for the diagnosis of gallbladder masses. Gastrointest Endosc. 2003;57:251–4.

28. Mallery S, Matlock J, Freeman ML. EUS-guided rendezvous drainage of obstructed biliary and pancreatic ducts: report of 6 cases. Gastrointest Endosc. 2004;59:100–7.

29. Kahaleh M, Yoshida C, Kane L, Yeaton P. Interventional EUS cholangiography: a report of 5 cases. Gastrointest Endosc. 2004;60:138–42.

30. Kahaleh M, Wang P, Shami VM, Tokar J, Yeaton P. EUS-guided transhepatic cholangiography: report of 6 cases. Gastrointest Endosc. 2005;61:307–13.

31. Kahaleh M et al. Interventional endoscopic ultrasound cholangiography: mid-term follow-up of 18 Cases. DDW 2005, W1226.

32. Poley JW et al. EUS-guided transbulbar rendezvous after unsuccessful ERCP. A report of 2 cases. DDW 2005, W1271.

33. Parasher VK, Hernandez LV, Leveen RF, Mladinich CR, Nonabur V, Bhutani MS. Lymph sampling and lymphangiography via EUS-guided transesophageal thoracic duct puncture in a swine model. Gastrointest Endosc. 2004;59:564–7.

34. Dewitt J, McHenry L, Fogel E, Leblanc J, McGreevy K, Sherman S. EUS-guided methylene blue pancreatography for minor papilla localization after unsuccessful ERCP. Gastrointest Endosc. 2004;59:133–6.

35. Will U, Meyer F, Manger T, Wanzar I. Endoscopic ultrasound-assisted rendezvous maneuver to achieve pancreatic duct drainage in obstructive chronic pancreatitis. Endoscopy. 2005;37:171–3.

36. Wiersema MJ, Wiersema LM. Endosonography-guided celiac plexus neurolysis. Gastrointest Endosc, 1996;44:656–62.

37. Hoffman BJ, Knapple WL, Bhutani MS et al. Treatment of achalasia by injection of botulinum toxin under endoscopic ultrasound guidance. Gastrointest Endosc. 1997;45:77–9.

38. Schiano TD, Fisher RS, Parkman HP et al. Use of high resolution endoscopic ultrasonography to assess esophageal wall damage after pneumatic dilation and botulinum toxin injection to treat achalasia. Gastrointest Endosc. 1996;44:151–7.

39. Van Dam J, Falk GW, Sivak MV et al. Endosonographic evaluation of the patient with achalsia: appearance of the esophagus using the echoendoscope. Endoscopy. 1995;27:185–90.

40. Miller LS, Liu J-B, Barbarevech CA et al. High-resolution endoluminal sonography in achalasia. Gastrointest Endosc. 1995;42:545–9.

41. Van Dam J. Endoscopic ultrasonography in achalasia. Endoscopy. 1994;26:792–3.

42. Birk JW, Khan AM, Gress F. The use of endoscopic ultrasound to evaluate response to intrasphincteric botulinum toxin in the treatment of achalasia. Gastrointest Endosc. 1998;47:AB141.

43. Kim JO, Hong SJ, Moon JH et al. High resolution endoscopic ultrasonography with miniature probes in achalasia. Gastrointest Endosc. 1998;47:AB148.

44. Catalano MF, Lahoti S, Alcocer E et al. Obliteration of esophageal varices using EUS guided sclerotherapy with color Doppler: comparison with esophageal band ligation. DDW 1998:3472.

45. Lahoti S, Catalano MF, Alcocer E, Hogan WJ, Geenen JE. Obliteration of esophageal varices using EUS-guided sclerotherapy with color Doppler. Gastrointest Endosc. 2000;51:331–3.

46. Lee YT, Chan FK, Ng EK et al. EUS-guided injection of cyanoacrylate for bleeding gastric varices. Gastrointest Endosc. 2000;52:168–74 .

47. Levy MJ, Louis M, WK Song et al. EUS guided angiotherapy of refractory gastrointestinal bleeding. Am J Gastroenterol. 2008;103:352–9.

48. Bhutani MS, Usman N, Shenoy V et al. Endoscopic ultrasound miniprobes-guided steroid injection for treatment of refractory esophageal strictures. Endoscopy. 1997;29:757–9.

49. Chang KJ, Nguyen PT, Thompson JA et al. Phase I clinical trial of allogeneic mixed lymphocyte culture (cytoimplant) delivered by endoscopic ultrasound-guided fine-needle injection in patients with advanced pancreatic carcinoma. Cancer. 2000;15:1325–35.

50. Hecht JR, Bedford R, Abbruzzese JL et al. A phase I/II trial of intratumoral endoscopic ultrasound injection of ONYX-015 with intravenous gemcitabine in unresectable pancreatic carcinoma. Clin Cancer Res. 2003;9:555–61.

51. Chang KJ, Lee JG, Holcombe RF, Kuo J, Muthusamy R, Wu ML. Endoscopic ultrasound delivery of an antitumor agent to treat a case of pancreatic cancer. Nat Clin Pract Gastroenterol Hepatol. 2008;5:107–11.

52. Gan SI, Thompson CC, Lauwers GY et al. Ethanol lavage of pancreatic cystic lesions: initial pilot study. Gastrointest Endosc. 2005;61:746–52.

53. Brugge WR. EUS guided pancreatic cyst ablation. Tech Gastrointest Endosc. 2007;9:46–50.

54. Jürgensen C, Schuppan D, Neser F, Ernstberger J, Junghans U, Stölzel U. EUS-guided alcohol ablation of an insulinoma. Gastrointest Endosc. 2006;63:1059–62.

55. Sahel J, Bastid C, Pellat B et al. Endoscopic cystoduodenostomy of cysts of chronic calcifying pancreatitis: a report of 20 cases. Pancreas. 1987;2:447–53.

56. Cremer M, Deviere J, Engelholm L et al. Endoscopic management of cysts and pseudocysts in chronic pancreatitis: long term follow up after 7 years of experience. Gastrointest Endosc. 1989;35:1–9.

57. Savides TJ, Gress F, Sherman S et al. Ultrasound catheter probe-assisted endoscopic cystogastrostomy. Gastrointest Endosc. 1995;41:145–8.

58. Binmoeller KF, Soehendra N. Endoscopic ultrasonography in the diagnosis and treatment of pancreatic pseudocysts. Gastrointest Endosc Clin N Am. 1995;5:805–16.

59. Gerolami R, Giovannini M, Laugier R. Endoscopic drainage of pancreatic pseudocysts guided by endosonography. Endoscopy. 1997;29:106–8.

60. Grimm H, Binmoeller KF, Sohendra N. Endosonography-guided drainage of a pancreatic pseudocyst. Gastrointest Endosc. 1992;38:170–1.

61. Etzkoran KP, DeGuzman LJ, Holderman WH et al. Endoscopic drainage of pancreatic pseudocysts: patient selection and evaluation of outcome by endoscopic ultrasonography. Endoscopy. 1995;27:329–33.

62. Chan AT, Heller SJ, Van Dam J et al. Endoscopic cystogastrostomy: role of endoscopic ultrasonography. Am J Gastroenterol. 1996;91:1622–5.

63. Wiersema MJ. Endosonography guided cystoduodenostomy with a therapeutic ultrasound endoscope. Gastrointest Endosc. 1996;44:614–17.

64. Fockens P, Johnson TG, van Dullemen HM et al. Endosonographic imaging of pancreatic pseudocysts before endoscopic transmural drainage. Gastrointest Endosc. 1997;46:412–16.

65. Catalano MF, Lahoti S, Geenen JE, Hogan WJ. Evaluation of pancreatic pseudocyst by EUS: can it determine by endoscopic modality treatment of choice? DDW, 1997:1067.

66. Giovannini M, Perrier H, Seitz JF. Cystogastrostomy entirely performed under endosonography guidance for pancreatic pseudocyst. DDW, 1997:631.

67. Norton ID, Clain JE, DiMagno EP et al. Endoscopic management of pancreatic pseudocyst by EUS localization of puncture site and balloon dilatation of fistulae. DDW, 1998:2253

68. Giovannini M, Pesenti C, Rolland AL, Moutardier V, Delpero JR. Endoscopic ultrasound-guided drainage of pancreatic pseudocysts or pancreatic abscesses using a therapeutic echo endoscope. Endoscopy, 2001;33:473–7.

69. Seifert H, Dietrich C, Schmitt T et al. Endoscopic ultrasound-guided one-step transmural drainage of cystic abdominal lesions with a large channel echoendoscope. Endoscopy. 2000;32:255–9.

70. Giovannini M, Bories E, Moutardier V et al. Drainage of deep pelvic abscesses using therapeutic echo endoscopy. Endoscopy. 2003;35:511–14.

71. Kahaleh M. EUS drainage of a mediastinal abscess. Gastrointest Endosc. 2004;60:158–60.

72. Seewald S. EUS-guided drainage of hepatic abscess. Gastrointest Endosc. 2005;61:495–8.

73. Wehrmann T. Endoscopic debridement of paraesophageal, mediastinal abscesses: a prospective case series. Gastrointest Endosc. 2005;62:344–9.

74. Matthes H. Endoscopic transgastric EUS guided drainage and necrosectomy of infected pancreatic pseudocysts. DDW, 2005.

75. Kahaleh M et al. Drainage of gallbladder fossa fluid collections with endoprosthesis placement under endoscopic ultrasound guidance: a preliminary report of two cases. Endoscopy. 2005;37:393–6.

76. Lee SS et al. EUS-guided transmural cholecystostomy as rescue management for acute cholecystitis in elderly or high-risk patients: a prospective feasibility study. Gastrointest Endosc. 2007;66:1008–12.
77. Giovannini M, Bories E et al. Hepaticogastrostomy by echoendoscopy as palliative treatment in patient with metastatic biliary obstruction. Endoscopy. 2003;35:1076–8.
78. Burmester E, Niehaus J, Leineweber T et al. EUS – cholangiodrainage of the bile duct: report of 4 cases. Gastrointest Endosc. 2003;57:246–50.
79. Mallery S, Matlock J, Freeman ML. EUS-guided rendezvous drainage of obstructed biliary and pancreatic ducts: report of 6 cases. Gastrointest Endosc. 2004;59:100–7.
80. Puspok A, Lomoschitz F, Dejaco C et al. Endoscopic ultrasound guided therapy of benign and malignant biliary obstruction: a case series. Am J Gastroenterol. 2005;100:1743–7.
81. Ponnudurai R, Giovannini M, Deviere J et al. EUS guided hepatico gastrostomy. Gastroenterol Endosc. 2004;58:AB4.
82. Kahaleh M, Hermandez AJ, Tokar J et al. Interventional EUS guided cholangiography: evaluation of a technique in evolution. Gastrointest Endosc. 2006;64:52–9.
83. Chan HH, Nishioka NS, Mino M et al. EUS-guided photodynamic therapy of the pancreas: a pilot study. Gastrointest Endosc. 2004;59:95–9.
84. Carrara S et al. Endoscopic ultrasound-guided application of a new hybrid cryotherm probe in porcine pancreas: a preliminary study. Endoscopy. 2008;40:321–6.
85. Pishvarian et al. EUS guided fiducial placement for cyberknife radiotherapy of mediastinal and abdominal malignancies. Gastrointest Endosc. 2006;64:412–17.
86. Jin Z et al. Endoscopic ultrasonography-guided interstitial implantation of iodine-125 seeds combined with chemotherapy in the treatment of unresectable pancreatic carcinoma: a prospective pilot study. Endoscopy. 2008;40:314–20.
87. Sun S et al. Endoscopic ultrasound-guided interstitial brachytherapy of unresectable pancreatic cancer: results of a pilot trial. Endoscopy. 2006;38:399–403.
88. Fritscher-Ravens A. Transgastric endo-surgical approaches to lymph nodes using EUS guidance. DDW. 2005, T1338.
89. Fritscher-Ravens A, Mosse CA, Mukherjee D et al. Transgastric gastropexy and hiatal hernia repair for GERD under EUS control: a porcine model. Gastrointest Endosc. 2004;59:89–95.
90. Fritscher-Ravens A, Ghanbari A, Cuming T et al. Comparative study on NOTES alone versus EUS guided NOTES procedures. Endoscopy. 2008;40:925–30.
91. Fritscher-Ravens A, Patel K, Ghanbari A et al. Natural orifice transluminal endoscopic surgery (NOTES) in the mediastinum: long-term survival animal experiments in transesophageal access, including minor surgical procedures. Endoscopy. 2007;39:870–5.
92. Ishikawa H et al. A comparison of image quality between tissue harmonic imaging and fundamental imaging with an electronic radial scanning echoendoscope in the diagnosis of pancreatic diseases. Gastrointest Endosc. 2003;57:931–6.
93. Hocke M et al. Contrast-enhanced EUS in discrimination between focal pancreatitis and pancreatic cancer. World J Gastroenterol. 2006;12:246–50.
94. Săftoiu A, Vilmann P, Popescu GL et al. Dynamic analysis of endoscopic ultrasound elastography used for the differentiation of benign and malignant lymph nodes. Gastrointest Endosc. 2007;66:291–300.
95. Săftoiu A, Vilmann P, Gorunescu F et al. Neural network analysis of dynamic sequences of EUS elastography used for the differential diagnosis of chronic pancreatitis and pancreatic cancer. Gastrointest Endosc. July 2008, epub ahead of print.
96. Vosburgh KG, Stylopoulos N, Estepar RS, Ellis RE, Samset E, Thompson CC. EUS with CT improves efficiency and structure identification over conventional EUS. Gastrointest Endosc. 2007;65:866–70.

Section V
Colon

Chair: R KIESSLICH and R SCHÖFL

8
Large bowel standards: quality, polyps, inflammatory bowel disease, stenoses, conventional chromoendoscopy

J. REGULA

QUALITY OF COLONOSCOPY

The issue of colonoscopy performance is currently of great concern for all important endoscopic societies and researchers. It is clear that the standard endoscopic examination of the large bowel should be of the highest possible quality. However, in recent years it has become clear that colonoscopy is often performed with suboptimal quality in clinical practice. Currently the process of defining quality requirements and quality parameters that should be monitored is underway. The five most important and most easily available quality parameters are: near-perfect bowel preparation, painless colonoscope insertion, high caecal intubation rate, perfect withdrawal technique allowing visualization of nearly all the surface of the bowel, and high adenoma detection rate. A full list of quality parameters and requirements is available elsewhere[1]. Endoscopic centres are currently supposed to monitor quality of the centre and quality of employed endoscopists. Special Quality Assurance Programmes should be introduced in all centres. In the simplest version quality can be provided if enough time is provided for each procedure, and if adenoma detection rate and caecal intubation rate are monitored.

POLYPS

The most frequent finding during colonoscopy is polyps. Although standards concerning polyps detection and polyps removal have been well defined for many years, still in some centres the practice concerning this issue is suboptimal. Several obvious rules should be remembered:

- All detected polyps should be removed; however, age of the patient and co-morbidities in order to avoid over-treatment should also be considered.

- Not all polyps must be removed endoscopically; there is a small fraction of polyps that are better managed surgically, and over-ambitious endoscopists should not insist on removing all of them.

- Endoscopists should know their abilities and limitations; they should know their endoscopic equipment, especially electrosurgical.

- All polyps should be retrieved for histology optimally to separate containers.

- Histologists should be provided with high-quality material, not destroyed, not cut into pieces.

- Completeness of removal should be assessed both endoscopically and histologically.

- Polypectomy should be performed in one piece, whenever possible.

- The six o'clock rule should be remembered (positioning of the polyp in the endoscopic view for removal).

- When cold snare polypectomy is performed there is no need for lifting the lesion; in fact lifting should not be done.

- When hot-snare polypectomy is done, coagulation current should be used whenever possible.

- Bowel should always be de-sufflated before polypectomy.

- Closing the snare for polypectomy should be optimally done by the endoscopist (and not by accompanying nurse).

The recommended decision tree concerning method of polyps removal is presented in Figure 1. Different centres can have slightly modified algorithms depending on the experience, availability of equipment and other factors.

Further therapeutic decisions depend on the histopathology report that should include: histopathological type of the polyp, dysplasia grade in case of adenomas and completeness of removal. The histopathological algorithm is presented in Figure 2.

Malignant foci within adenomas require more specific information, including: distance of cancer focus from dissection line, presence of lymphatic and blood vessels as well as cancer differentiation grade. If malignant foci are present within adenomas, endoscopic removal can be regarded as sufficient only if removal was not piecemeal and invasion was not deeper than 1000 µm into submucosa. Detailed information on this issue can be found elsewhere[2].

Patients in whom polyps have been removed need surveillance in the future. Recommendations concerning this step are changing recently in the direction of less intensive surveillance as compared to previous years. Recent recommendations are presented in Table 1. These recommendations are valid only if high-quality colonoscopy has been performed, the so-called 'clean colon' without polyps has been obtained and only if caecum was reached.

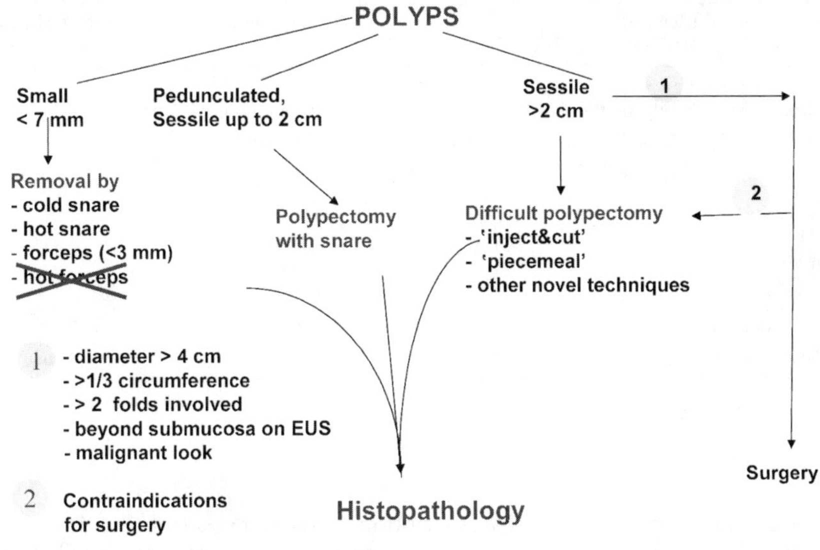

Figure 1 Decision tree for methods of removal of colorectal polyps

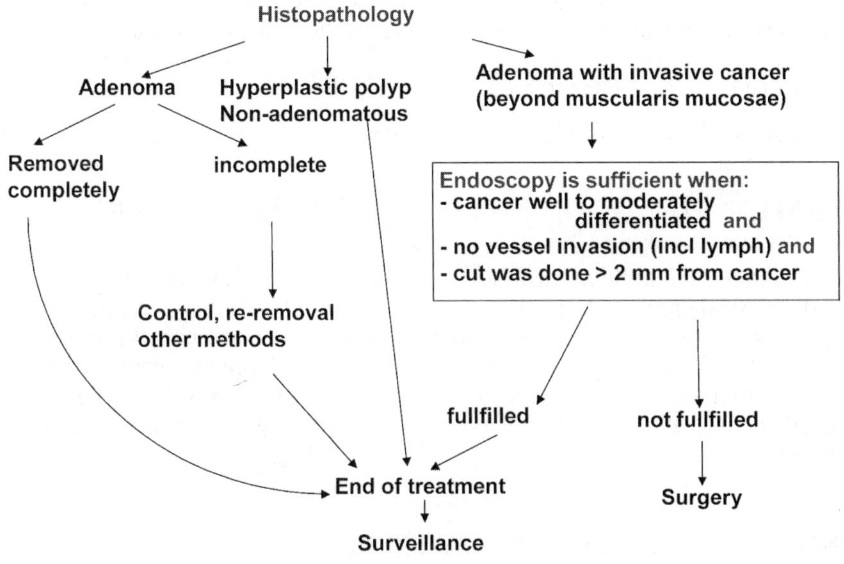

Figure 2 Algorithm of clinical decisions depending on histopathology reporting

Table 1 Recommendations concerning surveillance timing (time of the next control colonoscopy) after polypectomy providing that high-quality colonoscopy was performed and the so-called 'clean colon' has been obtained

Low-risk group	
Hyperplastic, rectal, small polyps	No surveillance
1 or 2 adenomas, less than 1 cm in diameter, tubular histology, low-grade dysplasia	5–10 years
Increased-risk group	
> 1 cm in diameter or high-grade dysplasia or villous component	3 years
3–10 adenomas all sizes	3 years
> 10 adenomas	< 3 years
Piecemeal or incomplete polypectomy	2–6 months until completeness ensured

Standards concerning polyp description have been well known for many years. Despite the fact that some endoscopists prefer to use the so-called free language, that should be discouraged. Polyp description should include its shape (pedunculated, sessile, flat), size (in centimetres), location (part of the colon or distance from anus on withdrawal of colonoscope), removal technique and whether endoscopic completeness was achieved. For shape description the Japanese classification can be used; it includes the following types:

- Protruding: Ip – pedunculated, Isp – semipedunculated, Is – sessile.

- Superficial: IIa – flat elevation, IIa +IIc – flat +depression, IIb – flat (no elevation).

- Depressed: IIc – mucosal depression, IIc + IIa – depression + edge.

Flat lesions are difficult to assess precisely and different definitions exist. Endoscopic definition states that it is a lesion with height less than half of the diameter; histological definition states that it is a lesion with thickness not greater than 2 times the thickness of adjacent normal mucosa measured from the muscularis mucosa to the top of the lesion. A special type of flat lesion is the so-called 'laterally spreading tumour'; these are really large, carpet-like flat lesions.

INFLAMMATORY BOWEL DISEASE (IBD)

The role of colonoscopy in IBD includes: providing diagnosis and differential diagnosis, assessment of the disease extent, defining the endoscopic activity, monitoring therapy especially mucosal healing after biologic therapy, and providing oncological surveillance in high-risk groups.

The following items should be observed during endoscopy and appropriately described: visibility of vascular pattern; presence of light reflexes (granularity); presence of ulcers or erosions and their shape, size and location; presence of contact bleeding to standard pressure usually with biopsy forceps; and presence of spontaneous bleeding. The standard description should mention continuity of involvement and list of diseased parts of the bowel.

There is no ideal scoring system in IBD. For ulcerative colitis the Baron modified score is used; however the interobserver variability is great with a kappa value of about 60% and the correlation with disease severity is poor. Another possibility often used in clinical trials is the Mayo endoscopic score, being a part of the general Mayo scoring system. The above scoring systems are far from ideal and are not standardized.

For Crohn's disease the situation is even more complicated. The oldest scoring system that is widely used is the CDEIS (Crohn's Disease Endoscopic Index of Severity)[3]. This scores severity in each anatomical segment of the bowel separately, and assesses the relative proportion of affected area, the relative proportion of severe lesions, and also adds extra points for such lesions as ulcerated stenoses. This system is reliable, reproducible and validated, and is currently regarded as gold standard. However, it is quite clear that it is complicated, time-consuming, with poor correlation to clinical activity and therefore not suitable for everyday clinical practice.

Recently, Daperno et al.[4] have proposed an easier and faster scoring system for Crohn's disease which applies 0–3 points for each of five ileocolonic segments. Four variables are assessed: presence of ulcers, ulcerated surface, affected surface and presence of narrowing. This score is called SES-CD (Simple Endocopic Score for Crohn's Disease) and is calculated as an algorithm, being a sum of points minus 1.4 times the number of affected segments.

A very important role of endoscopy in IBD (in both ulcerative colitis and Crohn's disease) is oncological surveillance because of cancer risk that is attributed to the long-lasting disease. Although recent studies seem to conclude that this risk is smaller than previously anticipated, the surveillance is still an important part of endoscopic practice. Recent ECCO recommendations[5] state that this surveillance should start 8–10 years after onset of ulcerative colitis to reassess disease extent. For those with extensive involvement, endoscopy is indicated every other year up to 20 years of disease and every year thereafter. Left-sided and distal colitis requires the start of regular surveillance 15 years after the onset of disease. Proctitis does not require surveillance. If primary sclerosing cholangitis (PSC) is associated with ulcerative colitis then surveillance should start at the moment of PSC diagnosis, and be performed annually.

During surveillance in IBD biopsies should be taken. Currently two alternatives are available. One is taking random biopsies – four every 10 cm plus targeted biopsies of any visible lesion. Another option, probably superior to random biopsies, is taking targeted biopsies during indigo carmine or methylene blue chromoendoscopy. This alternative method is reserved, however, to expert centres and expert endoscopists with appropriate experience.

Raised lesions encountered during surveillance endoscopy are clearly problematic for many endoscopists. The terminology issue is complicated, and confusion is observed due to different definitions used in different studies. It is difficult and complicated to define such lesions as dysplasia associated with a lesion or mass (DALM) and adenoma-like mass (ALM). Therefore, the author thinks it better to avoid these terms and just follow recent ECCO statements[5]: (A) a raised lesion with dysplasia should be completely resected; in the absence of dysplasia in the flat surrounding mucosa (at least four biopsies), meticulous endoscopic surveillance should be offered; (B) if resection is not possible, or if dysplasia is found in the surrounding flat mucosa, proctocolectomy should be recommended.

LARGE BOWEL STENOSES

It is now standard to balloon dilate anastomotic and IBD-related stenoses, and to stent or ablate malignant strictures. Although it is standard to decide about performing these procedures they are quite difficult, and require experience to provide efficacy and safety; these procedures should optimally be performed in referral centres.

Anastomotic stenoses occur in about 3–30% of colectomies. The preferred dilation system is TTS (through the scope) with the immediate and persistent success rate of about 70–90%. There are important practical clues about the size of the balloon that should first be employed, depending on the size of the opening; for pinhole stenosis a 12 mm balloon can be used, for <5 mm stenoses a 15 mm balloon can be used and for >5 mm stenoses a 18–20 mm balloon is used.

IBD stenoses should be treated only if symptomatic and if they are fibrotic and without active ulceration. Before the procedure the anatomy of the stricture should always be defined. The longer the stenosis the greater the risk of complications. Good and free endoscopic access should be provided for probable repeated procedures. Initial dilation should not exceed 10–15 mm. Some authors advocate triamcinolone injections into the stenoses after the successful dilation (40 mg + 5 ml saline). Early success is reported to be 81–95%, while late success goes down to 41–73%. Perforation as the most serious and frequent complication is described in 0–11% of patients. Large bowel stenting is indicated to palliate malignant stenosis or as a bridge to surgery. The success rate is reported to be 87–100%.

STANDARD LARGE BOWEL CHROMOENDOSCOPY

The main aim of using chromoendoscopy in the large bowel is to unmask contours and visualize borders of lesions detected. This method provides high-quality targeted biopsies and ensures endoscopic completeness of removal of flat lesions. The method also makes it possible to classify lesions according to the pit pattern and to predict histology. The clinical utility of this prediction is still debatable, but with the concurrent and routine use of additional methods such as high-resolution endoscopy and magnification, it may become quite useful in the future. The most popular staining agents are: 0.1–0.8% indigo carmine and 0.1% methylene blue.

Chromoendoscopy is becoming extremely useful for endoscopic surveillance in IBD patients with long-standing disease. So-called segmental chromoendoscopy, with segments of 20–30 cm stained for evaluation, will probably replace multiple random biopsies in that surveillance. Pancolonic staining that was tried in the past has not been proven to be of practical value.

References

1. Lieberman D, Nadel M, Smith RA et al. Standardized colonoscopy reporting and data system: report of the Quality Assurance Task Group of the National Colorectal Cancer Roundtable. Gastrointest Endosc. 2007;65:757–66.
2. Kudo S, Lambert R, Allen JI et al. Nonpolypoid neoplastic lesions of the colorectal mucosa. Gastrointest Endosc. 2008;68(4 Suppl.):S3–47.
3. Mary JY, Modigliani R. Development and validation of an endoscopic index of the severity for Crohn's disease: a prospective multicentre study. Groupe d'Etudes Thérapeutiques des Affections Inflammatoires du Tube Digestif (GETAID). Gut. 1989;30:983–9.
4. Daperno M, D'Haens G, van Assche G et al. Development and validation of a new, simplified endoscopic activity score for Crohn's disease: the SES-CD. Gastrointest Endosc. 2004;60:505–12.
5. Biancone L, Michetti P, Travis S et al. European evidence-based consensus on the management of ulcerative colitis: special situations. J Crohn's Colitis. 2008;2:63–92.

Section VI
Pancreas

Chair: A REPICI and GNJ TYTGAT

Section VII
Endoscopy in competition

Chair: R KIESSLICH and PN MEIER

9
Endoscopy in competition: diagnostics

D. HARTMANN

INTRODUCTION

Gastrointestinal endoscopy is one of the most important developments in medical diagnostics in the past century. Today, especially, radiological techniques are in competition with endoscopy.

Over recent decades the incidence of pancreatic cancer has increased. One of the most promising techniques for early detection of pancreatic lesions seems to be endoscopic ultrasound (EUS). In early studies EUS was superior or at least equal to other imaging modalities regarding sensitivity, determining tumour size and extent, lymph node involvement and vascular infiltration. With rapid advances in technology, computed tomography (CT) and magnetic resonance imaging (MRI) have achieved better results. The highest accuracy in assessing the extent of primary tumour, locoregional extension, vascular invasion, distant metastasis, tumour TNM (tumour–node–metastasis) stage and tumour resectability seems to be with helical CT, whereas EUS has the highest accuracy in assessing tumour size and lymph node involvement. For assessment of tumour resectability a combination of CT and EUS seems to be the procedure with the highest accuracy.

Magnetic resonance cholangiopancreatography (MRCP) plays an important role in the diagnosis of abnormalities of the pancreatic and biliary tract. In many cases, MRCP supplanted endoscopic retrograde cholangio-pancreatography (ERCP) and percutaneous transhepatic cholangiography (PTC) in the initial diagnostic evaluation and follow-up of diseases of the pancreas, gallbladder, and biliary tract. This is largely due to its non-invasive nature, avoiding possible complications that may occur with more invasive imaging such as pancreatitis or duodenal perforation, as well as the associated risks of sedation.

Virtual colonoscopy is based on CT or MRI three-dimensional data sets. Available large, prospective studies comparing CT colonography and conventional colonoscopy have shown a high per-polyp sensitivity. Despite promising results the future of CT colonography as a screening method remains uncertain, because potentially healthy people are exposed to considerable doses of ionizing radiation. Therefore, it seems reasonable to focus on MRI for colorectal cancer screening.

In summary, the radiological imaging methods are in competition with gastrointestinal endoscopy. These techniques are necessary for a better diagnostic work-up, especially in the staging of gastrointestinal malignancies.

EUS VERSUS CT

Diagnosis of pancreatic cancer

The incidence of pancreatic cancer has increased continuously over recent decades. Despite rapid improvements in imaging technologies and therapeutic modalities the prognosis remains poor. The overall 5-year relative survival rate for 1996–2002 is estimated to be 5.0%[1]. It seems to be even less, if data are critically reviewed. Carpelan-Holmström et al. collected slides or paraffin blocks from patients recorded as having histologically proven pancreatic ductal adenocarcinoma who survived for at least 5 years after diagnosis. They were re-evaluated in a double-blind fashion by three pathologists with special expertise in pancreatic pathology. In 26 patients recorded as having histologically proven pancreatic ductal adenocarcinoma, re-evaluation of histological specimens confirmed this diagnosis in only 10 patients. The adjusted 5-year survival rate for pancreatic ductal adenocarcinoma was 0.2%[2]. At the time of diagnosis about 20% of patients are meant to be candidates for curative resection, but only 7% of pancreatic cancers are found to be localized to the organ without locoregional spreading or distant metastases (AJCC stage 1) and, therefore, resectable in a curative intention. Even if they are found to be in stage 1, the prognosis remains poor, with a 5-year survival rate of 19.6%[1]. These data underline the importance of early diagnosis of pancreatic cancer, but pain, jaundice, weight loss and obstruction are usually late symptoms.

EUS

One of the most promising imaging techniques for early detection of pancreatic cancer is EUS. With its high resolution it is able to detect focal lesions as small as 2–3 mm with the possibility of obtaining tissue samples by fine-needle aspiration (FNA) or truecut needle biopsy for histopathological examination. There are three fundamentally different techniques of EUS available at present, each with pros and cons: (1) electronic or mechanical radial scanning scopes, in which the electronic scanning scopes seem to produce better B-mode image quality with no apparent difference in manoeuvrability, endurance and endoscopic images[3]; (2) linear scanning scopes; (3) radial or linear scanning probes for use with standard scopes or alone. Frequencies range from 5 to 20 MHz for scopes up to 30 MHz for probes. The accuracy in staging of pancreatic cancer is equivalent for radial and linear scanners[4], in which radial scanners offer a better overview of surrounding structures, whereas linear scanners allow the safe execution of tissue sampling. Indications for EUS, in

Table 1   Indications for EUS for detecting pancreatic tumours

Persistent epigastric and/or back pain
Acute onset of diabetes in the elderly
Unexplained weight loss
Acute or chronic pancreatitis
Suspect results in other imaging modalities
High-risk individuals (e.g. persons with a strong family history of pancreatic cancer,
with Peutz–Jeghers syndrome, or multiple endocrine neoplasia

Table 2   Results for accuracy of EUS for detecting pancreatic cancer

Reference	Accuracy (%)
Legmann et al.[6]	93
Akahoshi et al.[7]	94
Cannon et al.[8]	78
Ahmad et al.[9]	69
Meining et al.[10]	72
Soriano et al.[11]	63

relation to pancreatic cancer, are listed in Table 1. EUS has been described as a highly sensitive method, but results for accuracy, especially in the staging of pancreatic cancer, differ. Initial studies showed excellent accuracy up to 94%, but early euphoria flew away, and results in later publications declined (Table 2 and refs 5–11). Accuracy seems to be around 60–70%. If tissue diagnosis is necessary before therapy, EUS-guided FNA should be the method of choice. EUS-FNA is highly sensitive (84%), specific (97%), accurate (84%) and has a high positive predictive value (99%) with rare major complications, but negative predictive value is low with only 64%[12]. If pancreatic cancer is suspected, and if EUS-FNA is negative, cancer cannot be excluded, and operation will be the next step despite a positive or negative result in FNA.

Comparing EUS to other techniques

Early studies showed high sensitivity and accuracy for EUS, as mentioned above. Regarding sensitivity, determining tumour size and extent, lymph node involvement and vascular infiltration, EUS was superior or at least equal to other imaging modalities such as CT or MRI in most studies[6,13]. With rapid advances in technology CT and MRI have reached better results. Soriano et al. compared EUS with helical CT, MRI and angiography in a prospective study with histopathological or surgical confirmation of results[11]. When each imaging technique is looked at alone, helical CT reached the highest accuracy in assessing extent of primary tumour, locoregional extension, vascular invasion, distant metastasis, tumour TNM stage and tumour resectability, whereas EUS achieved the highest accuracy in assessing tumour size and lymph node involvement. A major problem in staging pancreatic cancer correctly is the prediction of resectability. The combination of CT and EUS proved to be the method with the highest accuracy compared to each single technique to predict tumour resectability. With regard to cost minimization, the combination of CT and EUS seems to increase the price compared with each single method. However, if cost of unnecessary explorative laparotomies was taken into account, the cost minimization analysis favoured a sequential strategy in which EUS was used as a confirmatory technique in those patients in whom helical CT suggested resectability of the tumour.

EUS is not a foolproof method. Even among experienced endosonographers there is high interobserver variation[14,15]. Furthermore, the accuracy of EUS seems to be dependent on additional clinical and imaging information[10]. Meining et al. retrospectively analysed EUS examinations/video tapes of 101 patients with resected tumours of the oesophagus, stomach and pancreas in three different ways: under routine clinical conditions, strictly blinded and in an unblinded fashion with additional information from endoscopic appearance (oesophagus, stomach) or CT (pancreas)[16]. The overall accuracy of T staging for pancreatic cancer was 72.2% and 75.0%, respectively, for routine and unblinded analysis, but only 61.1% for evaluation in a strictly blinded fashion. Additional possible associated factors that may increase the likelihood of a false-negative EUS examination are chronic pancreatitis, diffusely infiltrating carcinoma, a prominent ventral/dorsal split and a recent episode of acute pancreatitis[17].

CT or EUS in the detection of pancreatic cancer

Over recent decades the incidence of pancreatic cancer has increased continuously. The prognosis remains poor despite rapid improvements in imaging techniques and therapeutic modalities. EUS seemed to be one of the most promising techniques for early diagnosis. With or without FNA it has a high sensitivity, whereas accuracy in TNM staging differs. Optimistic results in early studies gave way to a more critical view. EUS, compared to CT, MRI and angiography, showed the highest accuracy in assessing tumour size and lymph node involvement, whereas helical CT had the highest accuracy in assessing extent of primary tumour, locoregional extension, vascular invasion, distant metastasis, tumour TNM stage and tumour resectability. The evaluation of tumour resectability should be done by a minimum of two imaging techniques, in which the combination of CT and EUS proved to be the method with highest accuracy at lowest cost.

ERCP VERSUS MRCP

MRCP

MRCP is a relatively recent advance in pancreaticobiliary imaging, originally introduced in 1991[18]. In many cases MRCP has supplanted ERCP and PTC in the initial diagnostic evaluation and follow-up of diseases of the pancreas and the biliary tract. This is largely due to its non-invasive nature, avoiding possible complications that may occur with more invasive imaging such as pancreatitis, duodenal perforation, haemorrhage, sepsis, as well as the associated risks of sedation. MRCP does not utilize ionizing X-ray radiation, as do ERCP or PTC, and does not require the same degree of operator skill or patient preparation. The ductal diameter is often more accurately portrayed as the duct is not artificially distended with administered contrast. The failure rate is also much lower than that for ERCP, being limited only by factors such as patient cooperation and ability to breath-hold.

MRCP has become the technique of choice in patients with factors contributing to a high failure rate for ERCP, such as oesophageal, gastric, or duodenal obstruction, stricturing or oedema of the ampulla of Vater, periampullary duodenal diverticuli, or postsurgical bowel reconstruction such as choledochoenteric or pancreaticoenteric anastomoses or gastro-jejunostomy[19]. MRCP is especially excellent at depicting ductal anatomy beyond an obstructing lesion, which is impossible to demonstrate by ERCP. MRCP is absolutely the test of choice in patients who have an incomplete or failed ERCP.

When MRCP is combined with traditional T1- and T2-weighted cross-sectional imaging sequences, as well as pre- and post-gadolinium contrast imaging, extraductal disease of the liver, pancreas, or porta hepatis can also be evaluated. Although MRCP lacks the direct therapeutic and pathological diagnostic advantages of ERCP, MRCP can preprocedurally guide these more invasive tests. MRCP also does not have as high a spatial resolution as ERCP, and thus may not detect the earliest of ductal abnormalities, especially in small peripheral ducts. It may also be difficult to distinguish malignant from benign causes of obstruction using MRCP alone (which is why MRCP is often combined with traditional contrast-enhanced MRI of the abdomen for evaluation of extraductal tissues.

Principles and techniques of MRCP

MRCP takes advantage of the inherent T2-weighted contrast that exists between intra-abdominal slow-flow fluid-containing structures and the background organs and soft tissues. Fluids in the biliary and pancreatic tree as well as the bowel have a much longer T2 relaxation time than adjacent soft tissues. As a result, heavily T2-weighted sequences will depict these structures with a much higher relative signal intensity compared to background organ parenchyma and adjacent fat (which have shorter relaxation times).

Promising variations on MRCP have recently been developed involving use of a stimulant to pancreatic juice excretion, to aid in ductal distension and visualization, as well as use of alternative contrast agents with biliary excretion. Both of these techniques add a functional component to the evaluation of the pancreatic and biliary tracts.

A few minutes prior to MRCP imaging of the pancreatic tree, administration of 0.2 µg/kg of secretin intravenously over the course of 1 min stimulates secretion of pancreatic fluids and bicarbonate from the exocrine glands, promoting pancreatic ductal distension[20]. This aids in demonstrating pancreatic ductal anatomy as well as in resolving whether cystic lesions of the pancreas communicate with the main or the side-branch pancreatic ducts (helpful in the differentiation of intraductal papillary mucinous neoplasmia (IPMN) and pseudocysts from cystic neoplasms). During the first 5 min post-injection, concomitant sphincter contraction also helps in distending the pancreatic ducts. Continued dynamic MRCP imaging over time may be performed to observe emptying of this pancreatic fluid into the duodenum to subjectively quantify pancreatic exocrine function and evaluate for sphincter of Oddi dysfunction[21,22]. As secretin is very well tolerated by most patients (with a low incidence of allergic reactions), the only drawback to this technique lies in the cost and availability of this agent.

Diseases of the biliary tract

MRCP is ideally suited to the detection of biliary calculi, especially in this age of routine laparoscopic cholecystectomy where surgery may prove difficult or may be complicated by the presence of bile duct stones. While ERCP is still considered the gold standard in evaluation of the biliary system, we deem MRCP to be comparable to ERCP in the detection of common bile duct stones and even more sensitive in the detection of intrahepatic ductal calculi.

Bile duct stones present as a round or ovoid filling defect creating a 'meniscus' margin with the proximal dilated bile duct. A major advantage of MRCP is its ability to depict the biliary system beyond an obstructing stone or calculus. In contradistinction, a stricture or obstructing mass will cause focal extrinsic narrowing of the bile duct. The presence of an obstructing mass rather than a stricture tends to cause a more focal and abrupt narrowing of the bile duct, with the appearance of 'shoulders' to the contours of narrowing.

In the diagnosis of common bile duct stones, MRCP achieves sensitivities of 80–100% and is thus superior to percutaneous sonography and CT imaging, and comparable to EUS[23–25]. Pitfalls in imaging, in addition to contraction of the sphincter of Oddi, include susceptibility artifact from adjacent surgical clips (i.e. cholecystectomy clips or prior gastrointestinal or pancreatic surgery), stents, bowel gas, or pneumobilia. These materials result in loss of signal in adjacent tissues (including fluid-filled ducts) which may simulate stone obstruction. Correlation to plain films and/or CT as well as comparison with gradient-echo images is often helpful in confirming the cause of this artifact. Pulsation artifact from adjacent vessels, biliary flow-related artifact, physiological compression from a crossing hepatic artery, as well as intraductal debris or blood, may also mimic stones.

MRCP can be helpful in the differentiation of strictures of the bile duct. In a prospective study, MRCP recognized benign stenosis with a sensitivity of 100% and malignant stenosis with a sensitivity of 91%. Additionally, MRCP (in contrast to ERCP) can identify the dilated bile duct beyond the stenosis and any other strictures[26]. In contrast, ERCP often shows only the bile duct below the stenosis. Furthermore, patients suffer the risk of cholangitis as a result of injecting too much contrast medium beyond the stenosis without subsequent immediate drainage.

Diseases of the pancreas

Detection of pancreatic cancer is the major interest in performing MR pancreatography in the evaluation of the pancreas and pancreas duct. A common finding at MRCP and ERCP is the 'double sign' in which both the pancreatic and common bile ducts are dilated. While this sign is sensitive and specific for pancreatic cancer (typically due to a mass at the head of the pancreas), this finding may be present in cases of focal pancreatitis of the pancreatic head as well as other benign causes of stricture. When there is a correlative clinical history of chronic pancreatitis or alcohol abuse, cancer and pancreatitis may be very difficult to differentiate. Findings that would suggest alcoholic chronic pancreatitis rather than cancer-causing ductal obstruction and dilation would be the presence of irregularity in the ductal wall and calibre as well as the presence of ductal calcification (often seen as filling defects in the duct). In a study of 124 patients a sensitivity of 83.3% with MRCP and 70.3% with ERCP was attained at comparable specificity in the detection of pancreatic cancer[27]. Factors crucial to evaluate in the setting of a suspected pancreatic cancer are any findings that may preclude surgical resection. These include vascular involvement of structures such as the coeliac axis or hepatic artery, superior mesenteric artery and vein, or portal vein.

Algorithm for triage to MRCP or ERCP

In patients with suspected pancreaticobiliary disease, ERCP should be reserved for those requiring therapeutic intervention. However, difficulty arises in identifying patients likely to require therapy in the early phase of diagnostic work-up. Parnaby et al. have developed an algorithm (Figure 1) based upon prospective assessment of ERCP patients for triage of patients to MRCP or ERCP with suspected pancreaticobiliary disease[28]. A total of 125 patients were stratified into different categories by clinical, ultrasound and liver function test findings. The algorithm stratified patients by the likelihood of therapeutic intervention. In summary, this study confirms that an algorithm-based approach can reproducibly predict those patients requiring therapeutic biliary intervention. Using an algorithm-based approach unnecessary MRCP and ERCP may be avoided, and the utilization of resources potentially optimized.

COLONOSCOPY VERSUS VIRTUAL COLONOSCOPY

Colorectal cancer screening

Colorectal cancer (CRC) remains the second leading cause of cancer death for both women and men[1], with more than 130 000 newly diagnosed cases and 50 000 deaths each year in the United States alone[29]. Most colon cancers develop from non-malignant colonic adenomas or polyps over a comparatively long time period ranging between 24 and 60 months[30]. Reflecting this adenomatous pathogenesis of most CRC, polyp screening with subsequent polypectomy has been shown to constitute an effective approach for

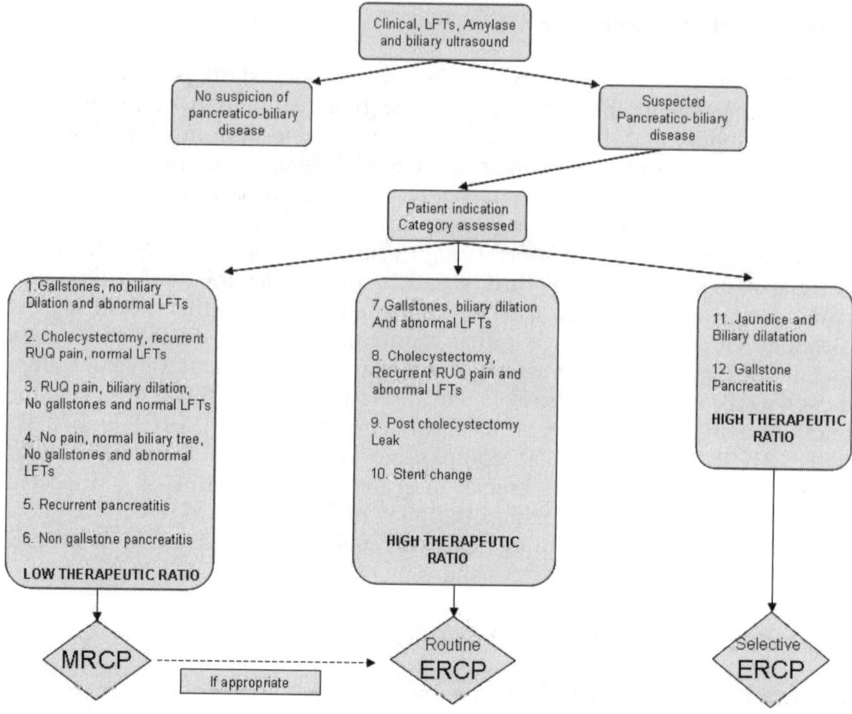

Figure 1 Algorithm for investigation by MRCP or ERCP[28] (LFT, liver function test; RUQ, right upper quadrant)

decreasing the incidence of this malignant tumour[31]. Thus, colorectal screening for polyps may be considered one of the most promising preventive measures in medicine.

Most available colorectal screening modalities, including testing for occult faecal blood or double-contrast barium enema, are associated with insufficient diagnostic accuracy[32,33]. Conventional optical colonoscopy has been established as an accurate method to examine the colon, with high sensitivity and specificity regarding the detection of colorectal polyps. Despite the availability of sufficient screening options, CRC remains a considerable cause of morbidity and mortality. This discrepancy between theoretical potential and clinical reality is caused mainly by poor patient acceptance, which reflects considerable procedural pain coupled with the rigours of preparatory bowel cleansing as well as the risk of complications such as perforations, and limits the acceptance of colonoscopy for CRC screening. Although there are various psychological factors inhibiting the acceptance of cancer screening programmes in general, efforts targeting the colon have been particularly problematic. Even in countries with free access to the diagnostic measure, participation in cancer screening programmes based on optical colonoscopy is suboptimal[33]. It has been shown that, even when offered free of charge, a huge majority of patients refused to undergo conventional colonoscopy for primary CRC screening. All these facts have motivated the development and evaluation of additional modalities to assess the large bowel, including virtual colonoscopy.

Virtual colonoscopy

Virtual colonoscopy (VC) is based on CT or MRI three-dimensional data sets. VC is not limited to endoscopic viewing. The three-dimensional data sets can be scrolled in a traditional two-dimensional mode on a workstation in any desired plane. This type of multiplanar reformation analysis depicts the colonic lumen and the colonic wall in relation to the surrounding abdominal morphology. Even in the presence of a stenotic tumour the entire colon can be assessed, which often is not possible in conventional colonoscopy. Another characteristic of VC is the possibility of simultaneously assessing all other abdominal organs within the displayed field of view. Especially in patients with CRC, the simultaneous assessment of the liver can be helpful for approving or excluding the presence of liver metastases.

Available large, prospective multicentre studies comparing CT colonography (CTC) and conventional colonoscopy have shown a wide variation in results[34–36]. Reasons for the variability reported in these studies include variation in the study population relative to the risk for neoplasia, variation in the techniques used to prepare the patients and perform the studies, differences in CTC technology, and variability in the manner in which CTC have been read. In the most important study using the latest techniques the per-polyp sensitivities were 86% and 92%, and per-patient sensitivities 89% and 94% for a cut-off size of 6–10 mm, respectively, comparable to conventional colonoscopy[34].

Despite promising results, the future of CTC as a screening method remains uncertain because potentially healthy people are exposed to considerable doses of ionizing radiation. The radiation issue may even evolve into a public health concern, because screening examinations of the colon should be repeated at regular intervals (every 3–5 years). Therefore, it seems reasonable to focus on MRI for CRC screening. The technique is not associated with any radiation exposure or other harmful side-effects. Furthermore, contrast agents applied in conjunction with MRI are characterized by a more favourable safety profile than CT contrast agents because they lack any nephrotoxicity and are associated with far fewer anaphylactoid reactions[37,38].

Magnetic resonance colonoscopy (MRC)

Technique

Before the examination, bowel preparation must be performed in a manner similar to that required for conventional colonoscopy, and patients should be screened for general contraindications to MRI, such as presence of metallic implants or severe claustrophobia. Hip prostheses, which are generally not considered a contraindication to MRI, may lead to strong artifacts in the region of the rectum and sigmoid colon and impede a sufficiently diagnostic image quality. Therefore, patients with hip prostheses should not be examined.

Similar to contrast-enhanced three-dimensional MR angiography, MRC is based on the principles of ultrafast imaging[39]. Because data acquisition must be performed under breath-holding conditions, the use of 1.5 T scanners equipped with strong gradient systems is mandatory. A combination of two large flex surface coils should be used for signal reception to ensure the coverage of the entire large bowel. A sufficient distension of the large bowel loops must be accomplished. In their physiological state most bowel segments are collapsed and cannot be depicted properly. Bowel distension must be achieved by administering distending media. Eventually, a high contrast between the bowel wall and the bowel lumen is important. Contrast mechanisms that allow an accurate display of the colonic wall depend strongly on the MR sequences applied and the use of intravenous and rectal contrast agents.

Diagnostic performance of MRC

In contrast to CTC, only limited data exist comparing MRC and conventional colonoscopy in the detection of colorectal polyps (Table 3). In a recent trial, MRC with the dark lumen technique was compared with conventional colonoscopy, which served as the standard of reference[40]. One hundred patients with different clinical indications were examined prospectively. MRC was followed by subsequent conventional colonoscopy for the same time period. Regarding data analysis, endoscopic and histological results were compared with MRC. In 49 patients, 107 colorectal masses were depicted by means of endoscopy. The sensitivity rate of MRC for adenomas on a per-polyp analysis was 100% for adenomas larger than 10 mm and 84.2% for adenomas between 6 and 9 mm in diameter. When using a per-patient analysis the overall sensitivity rate for the detection of colorectal masses was 90%. There were a few false-positive results, and specificity of MRC amounted to 96%. In summary, MRC showed a high accuracy for the detection of adenomas and carcinomas > 5 mm.

The outlined results were confirmed by other trials. In a recently published study 122 subjects with suspected colorectal disease (48 polyps) underwent 'dark lumen' MRC followed by conventional colonoscopy[41]. None of 30 polyps measuring ≤ 5 mm identified by conventional colonoscopy were detected on MRC images. In the 6–10 mm size group, MRC correctly detected 16 of 18 documented lesions on conventional colonoscopy. Additionally, two polyps ≥ 10 mm and all nine CRC were correctly seen on MRC images.

One major issue relates to the inability of MRC to detect colorectal masses < 5 mm. Small colorectal lesions will probably become detectable by MRC in the future. New technical refinements, including parallel acquisition techniques, will be implemented[42,43], and spatial resolution may be increased. Flat adenomas are likely to remain elusive, however.

Table 3 Studies comparing MRC and conventional colonoscopy

			Per-polyp sensitivity (%)		Per-patient sensitivity (%)		Per-patient specificity (%)	
Reference	Subjects (n)	Total lesions (n)	6–9 mm	≥10 mm	6–9 mm	≥10 mm	6–9 mm	≥10 mm
Lubold et al.[39]	132	189	61	96	Overall[†] 93		Overall[†] 99	
Pappalardo et al.[48][*]	70	130	96	100	Overall[†] 96		Overall[†] 93	
Ajaj et al.[41][**]	122	59 (9 carcinomas)	16/18 sensitivity: NR	11/11 sensitivity: NR	NR	NR	NR	NR
Hartmann et al.[40][**]	100	114 (7 carcinomas)	84 for adenomas	100 for adenomas	84 for adenomas	100 for adenomas	99 for adenomas	100 for adenomas

*Bright lumen MRC.

**Dark lumen MRC.

[†]Alternative category definition.

NR, not reported.

Indications for MRC

There are several proven indications for MRC. In patients with incomplete endoscopy caused by stenosis or elongated bowel segments, virtual colonoscopy (either based on MRI or CT) has been shown to provide useful additional information[44–47]. A recent trial evaluated the impact of MRC on patients who had undergone incomplete colonoscopy[44]. Thirty-two patients with incomplete endoscopy for different reasons (high-grade stenosis in 26 patients, extreme patient intolerance in one patient, and technical challenges associated with an elongated colon in five patients) underwent same-day dark lumen MRC. Of the 26 patients with high-grade stenosis, 19 underwent surgery with histopathological confirmation of the initial diagnosis. Follow-up colonoscopy was carried out in 14 patients with surgically treated stenosis. In six of these 14 patients, nine polyps identified at the initial MRC were confirmed and removed during a postoperative conventional colonoscopy.

There are still no data regarding the impact of MRC on CRC screening. Because most CRC develop over a period of several years from adenomatous polyps, this pathogenesis makes CRC to a large extent preventable. Detection and removal of polyps eliminate the risk of subsequent malignant degeneration. Implementations of screening programmes have been shown to reduce the incidence of CRC by more than 80%[31].

MRI includes all properties, which is necessary for a successful screening tool. The technique is not associated with any exposure to ionizing radiation and lacks any other known harmful side-effects. Because of its non-invasive character, patient acceptance is not negatively impacted. Although MRI has been found to be an accurate means for the depiction of relevant colorectal masses, we must be aware that these results were based on trials performed in preselected patient cohorts. Further studies are needed to evaluate the value or MRC in a screening population.

FUTURE DIRECTIONS FOR VC

Over the past decade major technological advances in MRI scanners have allowed the ability to scan patients faster, using thinner slices. This allows for improved quality of MRC examinations. Some research centres are currently evaluating alternative displays that allow viewing larger areas of the colonic surface at one time. A 'virtual pathology' view bisects the colon along its longitudinal axis, opening the colon so that it may be inspected like a surgical pathological specimen. The accuracy of these novel visualization methods needs to be determined.

Computer-aided detection (CAD) of colorectal lesions is also under investigation as a way to shorten interpretation times. Computer software that allows automated polyp detection is under development. These computer algorithms are typically based on a presumed hemispheric shape or curvature of polyps. Another area under investigation is the development of faecal and fluid tagging protocols. Because of the reluctance of some patients to undergo any form of cathartic preparations, we believe that validation of 'faecal tagging' for screening will be important to further increase compliance. However, there are several additional reasons why we believe that MRC without catharsis will not represent a singular solution. MRC should offer a same-day polypectomy for significant polyps detected at MRC. This 'one-stop' service requires only a single preparation. This practice would not be possible with a 'faecal tagging' approach, since patients requiring polypectomy for MRC-detected lesions would first need to undergo additional preparation prior to conventional colonoscopy. Such a 'one-stop' service will be possible only if there is excellent cooperation between radiologists and gastro-enterologists.

References

1. Ries LAG, Harkins D, Krapcho M et al. SEER Cancer Statistics Review, 1975–2003. Bethesda, MD: National Cancer Institute.
2. Carpelan-Holmström M, Nordling S, Pukkala E et al. Does anyone survive pancreatic ductal adenocarcinoma? A nationwide study re-evaluating the data of the Finnish Cancer Registry. Gut. 2005;54:385–7.
3. Niwa K, Hirooka Y, Niwa Y et al. Comparison of image quality between electronic and mechanical radial scanning echoendoscopes in pancreatic diseases. J Gastroenterol Hepatol. 2004;19:454–9.
4. Gress F, Savides T, Cummings O et al. Radial scanning and linear array endosonography for staging pancreatic cancer: a prospective randomized comparison. Gastrointest Endosc. 1997;45:138–42.
5. Rösch T. Staging of pancreatic cancer. Analysis of literature results. Gastrointest Endosc Clin N Am. 1995;5:735–9.
6. Legmann P, Vignaux O, Dousset B et al. Pancreatic tumors: comparison of dual-phase helical CT and endoscopic sonography. Am J Roentgenol. 1998;170:1315–22.
7. Akahoshi K, Chijiiwa Y, Nakano I et al. Diagnosis and staging of pancreatic cancer by endoscopic ultrasound. Br J Radiol. 1998;71:492–6.
8. Cannon ME, Carpenter SL, Elta GH et al. EUS compared with CT, magnetic resonance imaging, and angiography and the influence of biliary stenting on staging accuracy of ampullary neoplasms. Gastrointest Endosc. 1999;50:27–33.
9. Ahmad NA, Lewis JD, Ginsberg GG, Rosato EF, Morris JB, Kochman ML. US in preoperative staging of pancreatic cancer. Gastrointest Endosc. 2000;52:463–8.
10. Meining A, Dittler HJ, Wolf A et al. You get what you expect? A critical appraisal of imaging methodology in endosonographic cancer staging. Gut. 2002;50:599–603.
11. Soriano A, Castells A, Ayuso C et al. Preoperative staging and tumor resectability assessment of pancreatic cancer: prospective study comparing endoscopic ultra-sonography, helical computed tomography, magnetic resonance imaging, and angiography. Am J Gastroenterol. 2004;99:492–501.
12. Eloubeidi MA, Chen VK, Eltoum IA et al. Endoscopic ultrasound-guided fine needle aspiration biopsy of patients with suspected pancreatic cancer: diagnostic accuracy and acute and 30-day complications. Am J Gastroenterol. 2003;98:2663–8.
13. Rösch T, Braig C, Gain T et al. Staging of pancreatic and ampullary carcinoma by endoscopic ultrasonography. Comparison with conventional sonography, computed tomography, and angiography. Gastroenterology. 1992;102:188–99.
14. Fritscher-Ravens A, Knoefel WT, Krause C Swain CP, Brandt L, Patel K. Three-dimensional linear endoscopic ultrasound-feasibility of a novel technique applied for the detection of vessel involvement of pancreatic masses. Am J Gastroenterol. 2005;100:1296–302.
15. Ahmad NA, Kochman ML, Brensinger C et al. Interobserver agreement among endosonographers for the diagnosis of neoplastic versus non-neoplastic pancreatic cystic lesions. Gastrointest Endosc. 2003;58:59–64.
16. Meining A, Rösch T, Wolf A et al. High interobserver variability in endosonographic staging of upper gastrointestinal cancers. Z Gastroenterol. 2003;41:391–4.

17. Bhutani MS, Gress FG, Giovannini M et al. No Endosonographic Detection of Tumor (NEST) Study. The No Endosonographic Detection of Tumor (NEST) Study: a case series of pancreatic cancers missed on endoscopic ultrasonography. Endoscopy. 2004;36:385–9.

18. Wallner BK, Schumacher KA, Weidenmaier W, Friedrich JM. Dilated biliary tract: evaluation with MR cholangiography with a T2-weighted contrast-enhanced fast sequence. Radiology. 1991;181:805–8.

19. Adamek HE, Weitz M, Breer H, Jakobs R, Schilling D, Riemann JF. Value of magnetic-resonance cholangio-pancreatography (MRCP) after unsuccessful endoscopic-retrograde cholangio-pancreatography (ERCP). Endoscopy. 1997;29:741–4.

20. Hellerhoff KJ, Helmberger H 3rd, Rösch T, Settles MR, Link TM, Rummeny EJ. Dynamic MR pancreatography after secretin administration: image quality and diagnostic accuracy. Am J Roentgenol. 2002;179:121–9.

21. Matos C, Metens T, Devière J et al. Pancreatic duct: morphologic and functional evaluation with dynamic MR pancreatography after secretin stimulation. Radiology. 1997;203:435–41.

22. Cappeliez O, Delhaye M, Devière J et al. Chronic pancreatitis: evaluation of pancreatic exocrine function with MR pancreatography after secretin stimulation. Radiology. 2000;215:358–64.

23. Laokpessi A, Bouillet P, Sautereau D et al. Value of magnetic resonance cholangiography in the preoperative diagnosis of common bile duct stones. Am J Gastroenterol. 2001;96:2354–9.

24. Zidi SH, Prat F, Le Guen O et al. Use of magnetic resonance cholangiography in the diagnosis of choledocholithiasis: prospective comparison with a reference imaging method. Gut. 1999;44:118–22.

25. Calvo MM, Bujanda L, Calderón A et al. Role of magnetic resonance cholangio-pancreatography in patients with suspected choledocholithiasis. Mayo Clin Proc. 2002;77:422–8.

26. Adamek HE, Albert J, Weitz M, Breer H, Schilling D, Riemann JF. A prospective evaluation of magnetic resonance cholangiopancreatography in patients with suspected bile duct obstruction. Gut. 1998;43:680–3.

27. Adamek HE, Albert J, Breer H, Weitz M, Schilling D, Riemann JF. Pancreatic cancer detection with magnetic resonance cholangiopancreatography and endoscopic retrograde cholangiopancreatography: a prospective controlled study. Lancet. 2000;356:190–3.

28. Parnaby CN, Jenkins JT, Ferguson JC, Williamson BW. Prospective validation study of an algorithm for triage to MRCP or ERCP for investigation of suspected pancreatico-biliary disease. Surg Endosc. 2008;22:1165–72.

29. Landis SH, Murray T, Bolden S, Wingo PA. Cancer statistics 1998. CA Cancer J Clin. 1998;48:6–29.

30. O'Brien MJ, Winawer SJ, Zauber AG et al. The National Polyp Study. Patient and polyp characteristics associated with high-grade dysplasia in colorectal adenomas. Gastroenterology. 1990;98:371–9.

31. Winawer SJ, Zauber AG, Ho MN et al. Prevention of colorectal cancer by colonoscopic polypectomy. The National Polyp Study Workgroup. N Engl J Med. 1993;329:1977–81.

32. Ahlquist DA, Wieand HS, Moertel CG et al. Accuracy of fecal occult blood screening for colorectal neoplasia. A prospective study using Hemoccult and HemoQuant tests. J Am Med Assoc. 1993;269:1262–7.

33. Rex DK, Rahmani EY, Haseman JH, Lemmel GT, Kaster S, Buckley JS. Relative sensitivity of colonoscopy and barium enema for detection of colorectal cancer in clinical practice. Gastroenterology. 1997;112:17–23

34. Pickhardt PJ, Choi JR, Hwang I et al. Computed tomographic virtual colonoscopy to screen for colorectal neoplasia in asymptomatic adults. N Engl J Med. 2003;349:2191–200.

35. Cotton PB, Durkalski VL, Pineau BC et al. Computed tomographic colonography (virtual colonoscopy): a multicenter comparison with standard colonoscopy for detection of colorectal neoplasia. J Am Med Assoc. 2004;291:1713–19

36. Rockey DC, Paulson E, Niedzwiecki D et al. Analysis of air contrast barium enema, computed tomographic colonography, and colonoscopy: prospective comparison. Lancet. 2005;365:305–11.

37. Murphy KJ, Brunberg JA, Cohan RH. Adverse reactions to gadolinium contrast media: a review of 36 cases. Am J Roentgenol. 1996;167:847–9.

38. Prince MR, Arnoldus C, Frisoli JK. Nephrotoxicity of high-dose gadolinium compared with iodinated contrast. J Magn Reson Imaging. 1996;6:162–6.
39. Luboldt W, Bauerfeind P, Wildermuth S, Marincek B, Fried M, Debatin JF. Colonic masses: detection with MR colonography. Radiology. 2000;216:383–8.
40. Hartmann D, Bassler B, Schilling D et al. Colorectal polyps: detection with dark-lumen MR colonography versus conventional colonoscopy. Radiology. 2006;238:143–9.
41. Ajaj W, Pelster G, Treichel U et al. Dark lumen magnetic resonance colonography: comparison with conventional colonoscopy for the detection of colorectal pathology. Gut. 2003;52:1738–43.
42. Steidle G, Schäfer J, Schlemmer HP, Claussen CD, Schick F. Two-dimensional parallel acquisition technique in 3D MR colonography. Rofo. 2004;176:1100–5.
43. Griswold MA, Jakob PM, Heidemann RM, et al. Generalized autocalibrating partially parallel acquisitions (GRAPPA). Magn Reson Med. 2002;47:1202–10
44. Hartmann D, Bassler B, Schilling D et al. Incomplete conventional colonoscopy: magnetic resonance colonography in the evaluation of the proximal colon. Endoscopy. 2005;37:816–20.
45. Ajaj W, Lauenstein TC, Pelster G et al. MR colonography in patients with incomplete conventional colonoscopy. Radiology. 2005;234:452–9.
46. Gryspeerdt S, Lefere P, Herman M et al. CT colonography with fecal tagging after incomplete colonoscopy. Eur Radiol. 2005;15:1192–202.
47. Neri E, Giusti P, Battolla L et al. Colorectal cancer: role of CT colonography in preoperative evaluation after incomplete colonoscopy. Radiology. 2002;223:615–19.
48. Pappalardo G, Polettini E, Frattaroli FM et al. Magnetic resonance colonography versus conventional colonoscopy for the detection of colonic endoluminal lesions. Gastroenterology. 2000;119:300–4.

10
Endoscopy in competition: therapeutics

G. TRIADAFILOPOULOS

INTRODUCTION: GETTING A NEW IDEA ADOPTED

> *There is nothing more difficult to plan, more doubtful of success, nor more dangerous to manage than the creation of a new order of thingsWhenever his enemies have the ability to attack the innovator, they do so with the passion of partisans, while the others defend him sluggishly, so that the innovator and his party alike are vulnerable.*

Niccolò Machiavelli, The Prince (1513)

The prophetic words of Machiavelli sound so true today, in an era of enormous scientific and technological innovation that has ushered the field of medicine so quickly forward. Endoscopy, in the 'baby boom' era of its growth, has been one of the many areas of innovation with individuals and teams of inventors and investigators working feverishly to accomplish and materialize new ideas. Such activity has created not only intellectual challenges for the innovators but also fierce competition to 'hit' the market first, to prevail and to profit. Yet, ultimately, the gain has been with the patients who have benefited from the fruits of such activity albeit, rarely, at the cost of unexpected untoward adverse events. Nevertheless, particularly in the field of therapeutic endoscopy – that is the subject of this chapter – the gains have far outweighed the losses, and gastroenterology, as a specialty, will never be the same because of the advances and promises that such innovation has brought forward.

Gastrointestinal endoscopy can be broadly viewed as two main but interdependent entities: 'diagnostic' and 'therapeutic'. The former typically has had to compete or enhance gastrointestinal imaging and other laboratory-based studies in the evaluation and the diagnostic assessment of disease. The latter, instead, has mostly served as a facilitator – not a competitor – to interventional radiology techniques and surgery, depending on the specific and individual needs. Figure 1 outlines the interdependence of these disciplines to each other and how each, and collectively, they can affect the care of a patient with gastrointestinal diseases.

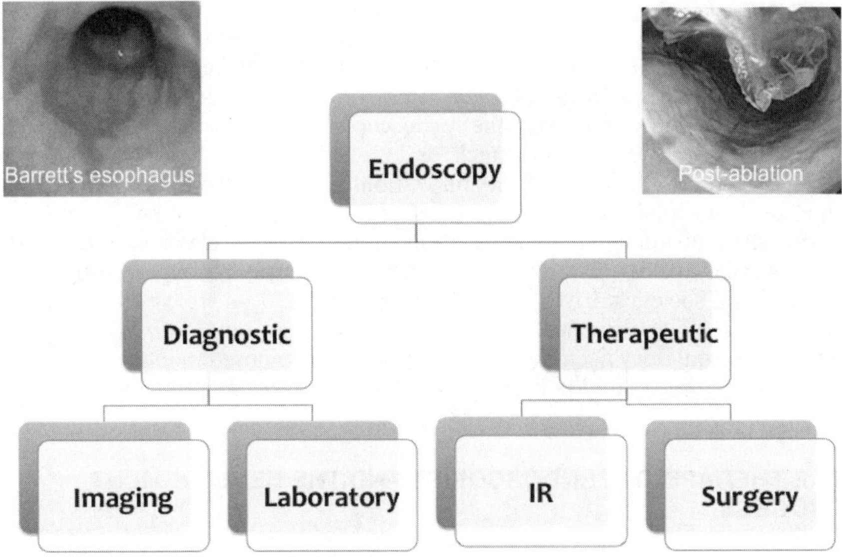

Figure 1 Interdependence of the various disciplines involved in the management of a patient with a gastrointestinal illness

ENDOSCOPIC INNOVATION

Endoscopic innovation could be seen as the idea, practice, or object that is 'perceived' as 'new' by practising endoscopists who will ultimately adopt it. Such innovation has to have the following attributes: relative advantage(s) to existing technologies, compatibility both with existing equipment and clinical values; acceptable complexity that will allow easy understanding and application to everyday use; trialability, that is, the opportunity to be tried hands-on; and visibility, that implies the ability to provide an almost immediate visible or palpable clinical effect, such as quick haemostasis, stricture palliation, etc. Recent examples of therapeutic innovations in endoscopy are: endoscopic mucosal resection (EMR), endoscopic antireflux therapies, radiofrequency ablation of Barrett's oesophagus, endoscopic submucosal dissection (ESD), endoscopic drainage of pancreatic cysts or collections, enteral stenting, endoscopic ultrasound (EUS)-guided intralesional chemotherapy. Natural orifice trans-endoscopic surgery (NOTES), has been the most recent development and is poised to become the next frontier in endoscopy.

THE DIFFUSION PROCESS

In general, any innovation, including a therapeutic endoscopic one, is communicated and adopted over time among various parties, such as industry, insurers, consumers (i.e. endoscopists), and ultimately to patients. Such adoption and ultimate quick or late diffusion may vary enormously, depending on the specifics of the innovation and the relative acceptance, over time, of the technology. Adopting endoscopic innovation could be: (1) *optional*, that is, the individual patient decides and adopts, typically electively and mostly on a self-pay basis; (2) *collective*, where a consensus among endoscopists/ professional societies drives adoption, typically based on strong evidence that supports but does not necessarily mandate its use; or (3) *authority-driven*, where the regulatory agents/government or payer-imposed mandates, as is the case of colonoscopy and polypectomy in patients over 50 years of age.

THE THERAPEUTIC ENDOSCOPIST AND THE DEVELOPMENT PROCESS

The therapeutic endoscopist is generally but variably involved in the development process of the innovation. Early on, the endoscopist is the one who identifies the needs and problems to be addressed and conducts experiments or advises on the research needed. The therapeutic endoscopist mostly plays a minor role in the development process of the innovation and is even less involved in its commercialization. Nevertheless, it is the endoscopist who will adopt and diffuse the technology and demonstrate – over time – its results and impact.

EVER-SHIFTING ENDPOINTS

The process of therapeutic innovation starts with the identification of the need, the definition of endpoints (clinical or surrogate); introduction of utilities, or measures of assessment; the assessment of comparative efficacy; safety evaluation; cost-effectiveness; and reimbursement. As an example, in the case of a novel endoscopic therapy for reflux, the need to treat gastro-oesophageal reflux disease non-invasively ignites the process, followed by the definition of the endpoints we are trying to address (symptom control, healing of oesophagitis, pH control, enhancement of the antireflux barrier, among others), then by utilization of well-designed means of assessment (i.e. questionnaires, endoscopy, pH monitoring); then the comparative assessment of the endoscopic approach over placebo or sham therapy or even fundoplication. Indispensable are the assessment of the frequency and severity of adverse events and eventually, if the innovation is going to succeed, the documentation of the technology's cost-effectiveness, since its ultimate fate will depend on it, given a very tight fiscal reimbursement environment.

THINKING OUTSIDE THE BOX

Thinking outside the box is a requirement for endoscopic innovation. The therapeutic endoscopist – usually as a member of the research and development team – should maintain hands-on practice with the innovation and be vigilant of the needs and problems encountered with the increasing use of the prototype equipment or device. Further, reassessment of norms based on an interactive attitude and dialogue with other members of the development team is pivotal. Synergy and mutual understanding are essential in the final delivery of a practical innovation or device that would have the best chances for success in clinical practice.

THE PRESENT: SYNERGY OR ANTAGONISM?

In modern, open-minded and experienced units around the world, therapeutic endoscopy has established its role not as a 'competitive' element to surgery or interventional radiology but as an essential partner in health-care delivery in a coordinated interdisciplinary way. This is taking place mostly in a fiscally independent fashion but it could in the future evolve into an even more efficient model of fiscally interdependent approaches, based on experience, new paradigms, cost-effectiveness assessment and guideline development. This way, a patient with a gastrointestinal illness will be seen by all members of the

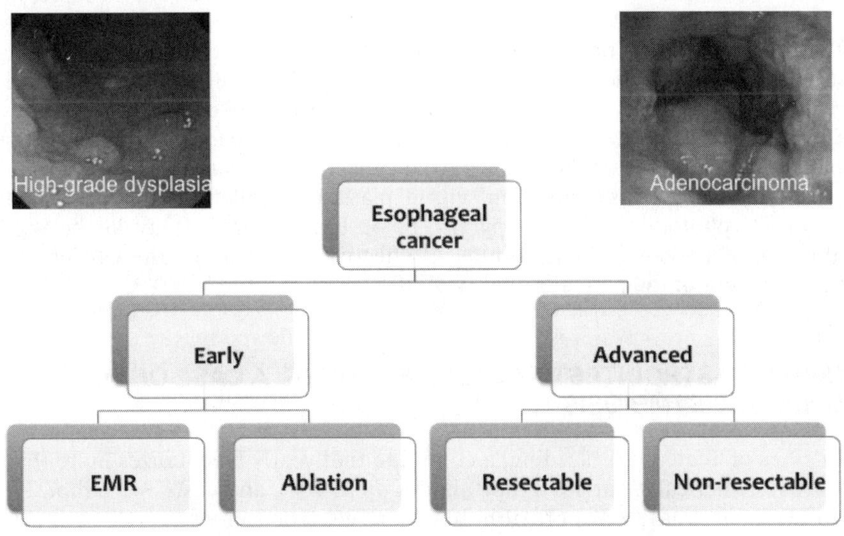

Figure 2 Example of algorithmic approach to oesophageal cancer

medical, radiological and surgical teams, who individually will assume their task demanded by a pertinent protocol set in place. Such collective experience, based on individual pathways of care, will ultimately allow all members of the team to evaluate their outcomes and adjust practices as needed for future implementation. Figure 2 exemplifies this issue with the case of oesophageal cancer. If the disease is detected early, before invasion, mucosal ablation and/ or endoscopic mucosal resection (EMR) are applied; in contrast, in advanced cases, resectability, determined by imaging studies, will define the need to proceed with surgery or chemoradiation or both. Furthermore, as exemplified in the case of nodular dysplasia in Barrett's oesophagus, EMR, performed early, is both a diagnostic and a therapeutic tool and is usually adequate for high-grade intra-epithelial neoplasia. The procedure, however, can be followed by surgical resection if the lateral or, more so, the deep margins are involved by invasive neoplasia. In contrast, if the margins were clear, a follow-up mucosal ablation of the surrounding Barrett's metaplasia using radiofrequency or cryotherapy would be adequate and curative.

In the case of high-grade intraepithelial neoplasia in patients with Barrett's oesophagus, the event is non-urgent and mostly outpatient; it has a higher prevalence in the elderly who carry higher morbidity and mortality; and it allows elective scheduling. Nevertheless there is some uncertainty with completeness post-EMR or ablation, while surgical morbidity and mortality are improving and resective surgery is often satisfying and definitive. Therefore, such conditions allow the luxury of a clinical and multidisciplinary debate and an improved clinical practice, based on collective experience that considers – on an equal basis – the respective roles of therapeutic endoscopy and surgery.

In cases of advanced, yet resectable, oesophageal cancer, 'bridging' during the pre-, peri-, and postoperative periods using self-expanding metal stents (SEMS) aims at relieving dysphagia, reducing the likelihood of aspiration, closing tracheo-oesophageal fistulas, allowing for neo-adjuvant chemotherapy to be delivered and may even cover treating post-operative leaks. In the palliation of non-resectable oesophageal cancer, self-expanding stents (metal/ plastic), Nd:YAG laser ablation, argon plasma coagulation (APC), ethanol injection, photodynamic therapy (PDT) or brachytherapy may all be used alone in a tandem fashion, aiming at effective palliation of the cancer and improvement of the patient's quality of life.

UPPER GASTROINTESTINAL (UGI) BLEEDING: A CASE OF MEDICAL-SURGICAL SYMBIOSIS

In cases of acute UGI bleeding, a condition that yearly hospitalizes more than 400 000 Americans, carries a mortality of up to 10%, and costs ~2 billion US dollars per year, cooperation between gastroenterology (therapeutic endoscopy) and surgery is more clear and validated. Figure 3 shows an algorithm of care of a patient with non-variceal UGI bleeding where combined medical and endoscopic therapies with intravenous acid suppression therapy, in conjunction with endoscopic haemostasis using various thermal or other haemostatic devices, are used. With this approach

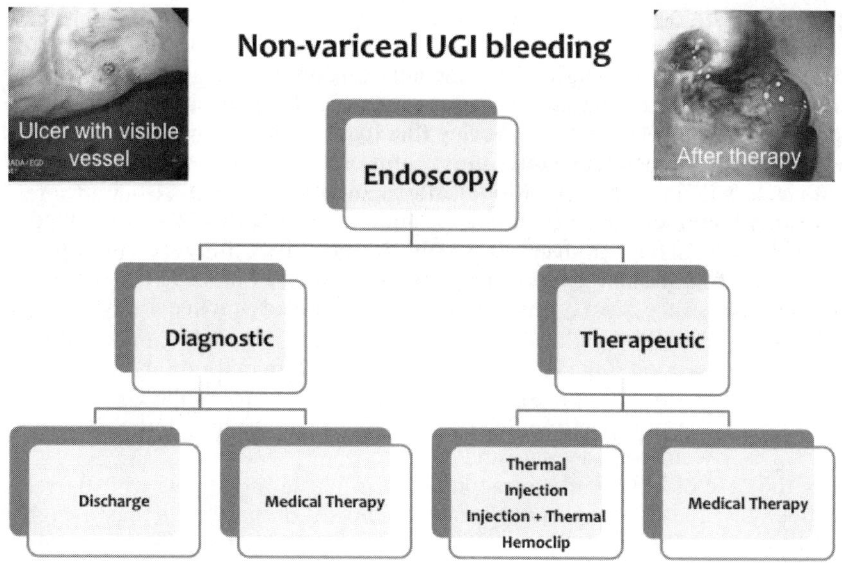

Figure 3 Example of a pathway followed in the diagnosis and management of a patient with upper gastrointestinal bleeding. Surgery is used only for failures of combined medical and endoscopic management

every UGI bleeding patient is first treated endoscopically and only if failure occurs does surgery become an option. This is mostly because, despite similar lengths of stay, amounts of blood transfusions required, or even 30-day mortality rates, complication rates after surgery are twice as large as with endoscopic therapy.

The decision between surgery versus therapeutic endoscopy for UGI bleeding is also based on the fact that the event is typically urgent, unpredictable, and mostly self-limited. UGI bleeding also has higher prevalence in the elderly, typically of higher morbidity and mortality risk, and there is also the need for immediate intervention. Under such conditions the operating room's schedule rigidity, and the more ready availability of endoscopy that can be done in the emergency or intensive-care unit setting, simplify the decision further. Surgical morbidity and mortality are high and surgery is often complex and unsatisfying. Here, the pendulum clearly favours endoscopic intervention first, then surgery, only for failures.

THE FUTURE

With the increasing complexity of medical care in an ageing population, the concept of integrated digestive diseases centers (IDDC) appears very appealing for the future. These centres will bring therapeutic endoscopy and surgery into a fiscally interdependent state, algorithms will be followed and improved outcomes will be expected. Modifications of practices will also be easy to implement and examine in terms of success or failure, but also of cost-effectiveness. The opportunities and potential of flexible therapeutic endoscopy in a milieu of laparoscopic surgery, as well as NOTES, will bring down barriers very quickly and change current clinical practice for ever.

11
State-of-the-Art Lecture:
Future perspectives: intraluminal endoscopy

J. F. RIEMANN and L. HELMSTADTER

Within recent decades gastrointestinal (GI) endoscopy has changed from a pure diagnostic tool to an incresead therapeutic discipline. GI endoscopy is replacing surgical interventions and has led, for example, to a paradigm change in the therapy of common bile duct stones including endoscopy sphincterotomy.

Up to now the main field of GI endoscopy has focused on palliative therapy (e.g. drainage procedures and stents). Today GI endoscopy is increasingly used under certain circumstances in the therapy of early cancer stages or in the case of precancerous lesions in the oesophagus, stomach and colon.

One of the main reasons for this development is technical progress. At this time new technologies allow excellent detection possibilities of suspected mucosal lesions. This progress is characterized by structure enhancement, high-definition television (HDTV), computerized virtual chromoendoscopy (narrow-band imaging, NBI), Fuji Intelligent Color Enhancement (FICE and I-Scan), the adapted haemoglobin index with measurement of the haemoglobin concentration of the mucosa and autofluorescence endoscopy. All are demonstrating so-called 'red-flag' techniques.

The history of small bowel diagnostics started with the first use of endoscopes in the early 1970s[1] followed by intraoperative endoscopy[2], transnasal sonde enteroscopy[3] and push enteroscopy[4]. The 21st century has now produced further new techniques such as capsule endoscopy (PillCam)[5], endocapsule[6] and balloon enteroscopy (double balloon[7,8], single balloon[9]).

These innovations are standard in most endoscopy centres, because they offer a significant simplification and improvement of examination techniques. They provide inspection of the entire small bowel with high diagnostic sensitivity and optional therapeutic interventions. Another technical success are small-calibre endoscopes such as the SpyGlass system for endoscopy of the pancreatic and common bile duct. The SpyGlass system consists of an endoscopy system with a 4-way direction possibility, independent rinsing channels and diagnostic and therapeutic options with single-use and multiple-use components.

One of the major aspects of future GI endoscopy is preventive medicine. Colorectal cancer is increasing worldwide. In Germany the numbers of screening colonoscopies do not increase despite the fact that neoplasias of the GI tract can be detected at very early stages. Reasons for the moderate acceptance of screening investigations are a lack of information and knowledge, but also fear of the examination itself. Improved instruments and new technologies could lead to a higher acceptance of screening examinations. New and promising techniques are arising: the CathCam system, the colonoscope with a guidewire[10], the ColonoSight system with a new single-use device[11], as well as the Invendo colonoscopy system which has a complete hydraulic single-use system[12]. Another innovation is the so-called Aero-O-Scope, a self-propelling and self-navigating colonoscopy system which moves due to CO_2 insufflation and allows a 360° view[13]. One of the most promising techniques may be the NeoGuide system, which consists of a computerized, partially automatic colonoscope with 64 guided segments and infrared probes, which will prevent loop formation, the existence of pain and complications[14]. Another new technique is capsule endoscopy[15,16] which, after the finalization of a pilot study in three German centres (Dusseldorf, Hamburg, Ludwigshafen) in 2008, will probably come to the market.

Virtual colonoscopy has also been developed further, and seems to be a true alternative to conventional colonoscopy in terms of screening procedures. Computed tomography colonoscopy has a sensitivity up to 89% (polyps 6–9 mm) and 94% (polyps > 10 mm) and a specificity of 80% (polyps 6–9 mm) and 96% (polyps < 10 mm) respectively[17]. A pilot study with magnetic resonance colonoscopy demonstrates comparable results with a sensitivity of 84% for 6–9 mm polyps and 100% for polyps < 10 mm[18]. Further results will come from the LUVIK study, a German multicentre study which has begun recently.

In the future a steady increase of examinations for palliation of malignant strictures may play a prominent role. New, self-enfolding metal stents (SEMS) with a radioactive iodine-125 layer can be placed in the oesophagus[19]. Partially double-layered, self-expanded Nitinol stents may be introduced in malignant gastroduodenal stenoses[20]. Radioactive palladium-103 stents[21], as well as self-expanding naturally degrading PLLA stents[22] and stents with Paclitaxel-eluding membrane[23,24] for the common bile duct are new therapeutic modalities in stenoses of the GI tract.

New endoscopic techniques such as endoscopic pyloroplasty[25] or submucosal endoscopic oesophageal myotomy are up-coming[26]. One of the most impressive new methods is endoscopic submucosal dissection (ESD), in which new and interesting instruments have been introduced, the ERBE Hybrid-Knife being one of these, which allows injection of fluids into the submucosa with simultaneous water jet dissection. Interesting also is the Olympus R-scope, which provides new modalities for these up-coming techniques.

Endoscopic ultrasound (EDS) is being increasingly used. New techniques consist of constructing an enteral anastomosis[27], transgastral lymph adenectomies[28] and transoesophageal operations on the heart[29].

Transluminal endoscopic interventions can be done only if sewing systems are at hand which allow the closing of the enterotomy. The so-called natural orifice transluminal endoscopic surgery (NOTES) procedures are one of the major challenges in the future when, after opening all the intestinal layers, these holes have to be closed. Instruments such as the Eagle Claw, the Double T-Bar (Olympus Medical) or the so-called g-Prox-system (USGI Medical) seem to be suitable for these procedures, and probably in the near future can be used economically.

Technical success, and the increasing invasiveness of endoscopic interventions require interdisciplinarity, e.g. procedures in the process of NOTES, endopathology with endocytology and endomicroscopy or the so-called rendezvous techniques which lead to new dimensions of interdisciplinary tumour therapy. Interdisciplinary endoscopic units, competence centres and the cooperation of various medical societies and groups are necessary, using common guidelines.

Endomicroscopy and endocytology, in combination with molecular imaging, will lead to endopathology. NOTES technology, which makes interdisciplinarity evident, will simplify interventions with a rapid re-creation, low pain and an increased healing process without infections of the peritoneum. In addition, there are no cosmetic changes. Due to these advantages, a worldwide variety of working groups have been initiated, for instance NOSCAR, EURO-NOTES and D-NOTES. Conventional endoscopes with a maximum flexibility have been constructed. New instruments such as the NeoGuide NOTEScope with a multi-tasking platform or a direct-drive system[30] are being tested at this time, with promising results.

A further future aspect of endoscopy will be endoscopic research. Supported by the industry and by scientific organizations for prospective studies, outcome research will change gastroenterological endoscopy.

Due to the increasing use of invasive techniques quality management of endoscopy will become more and more important. This can be achieved with standardized training procedures in certain training camps (GATE, ENDOAkademie) using improved simulators, quality controls (e.g. EPT register) and more transparency in documenting complications.

In conclusion one can say that, in the future, the main fields of endoscopy in gastroenterology will focus on technology, prevention, increasing invasivity, interdisciplinarity, research and quality management. This will lead to the fact that diagnostic sensitivity will increase, new therapeutic dimensions will arise and more research activities will give us a steadily growing consciousness for quality.

References

1. Classen M, Fruhmorgen P, Koch H. Demling L. [Fiberoptics endoscopy of the jejunum and ileum). Dtsch Med Wochenschr. 1972;97:409–11.
2. Bosseckert H, Schramm H, Lungershausen G. Machnik G. Oral intraoperative enteroscopy for diagnosis of multiple jejunal ulcers. Endoscopy. 1981;l3:7–18.
3. Tada M, Shimizu S, Kawai K. A new transnasal sonde type fiberscope (SSIF type VII) as a pan-enteroscope. Endoscopy. 1986;16:121–4.
4. Benz C. Martin WR, Arnold J, Jakobs R, Riemann JF. [Endoscopic study of the mall intestine with push enteroscopy. A prospective study]. Dtsch Med Wochenschr. 1997;122:391–5.

5. Iddan G, Meron G, Glukhovsky A, Swain P. Wireless capsule endoscopy. Nature. 2000;405:417.

6. Hartmann D, Eickhoff A, Damian U, Riemann JF. Diagnosis of small-bowel pathology using paired capsule endoscopy with two different devices: a randomized study. Endoscopy. 2007;39:1041–5.

7. Yamamoto H, Sekine Y, Sato Y et al. Total enteroscopy with a nonsurgical steerable double-balloon method. Gastrointest Endosc. 2001;53:216–20.

8. May A, Nachbar L, Wardak A, Yamamoto H, Ell C. Double-balloon enteroscopy, preliminary experience in patients with obscure gastrointestinal bleeding or chronic abdominal pain. Endoscopy. 2003;35:985–91.

9. Hartmann D, Eickhoff A, Tamm R, Riemann JF. Balloon-assisted enteroscopy using a single-balloon technique. Endoscopy. 2007;39(Suppl.1):E276.

10. Fritscher-Ravens A, Fox S, Swain CP, Milla P, Long G. CathCam guide wire-directed colonoscopy: first pilot study in patients with a previous incomplete colonoscopy. Endoscopy. 2006;38:209–13.

11. Shike M, Repici A, Cohen LB, Goldfarb-Albak S, Fireman Z. Major advances in colonoscopic technology: the ColonoSight®, a pull-power assisted disposable, non fiber-optic colonoscope. Gastrointest Endosc. 2004;59:113.

12. Roesch T, Adler A, Wiedenmann BH, Hoepffner N. A prospective pilot study to assess technical performance of a new single use colonoscope with inverted sleeve technology. Gastrointest Endosc. 2007;65:AB340.

13. Vucelic B, Rex D, Pulanic R et al. The Aer-O-Scope: proof of concept of a pneumatic, skill-independent, self-propelling, self-navigating colonoscope. Gastroenterology. 2006;130:672–7.

14. Eickhoff A, van Dam J, Jakobs R et al. Computer-assisted colonoscopy (the NeoGuide endoscopy system): results of the first human clinical trial ('PACE study'). Am J Gastroenterol. 2007;102:261–6.

15. Eliakim R, Fireman Z, Gralnek IM et al. Evaluation of the PillCam colon capsule in the detection of colonic pathology: results of the first multicenter, prospective, comparative study. Endoscopy. 2006;38:963–70.

16. Schoofs N, Deviere J, Van Gossum A. PillCam colon capsule endoscopy compared with colonoscopy for colorectal tumor diagnosis: a prospective pilot study. Endoscopy. 2006;38:971–7.

17. Pickhardt PJ, Choi JR, Hwang I et al. Computed tomographic virtual colonoscopy to screen for colorectal neoplasia in asymptomatic adults. N Engl J Med. 2003;349:2191–200.

18. Hartmann D, Bassler B, Schilling D et al. Colorectal polyps: detection with dark-lumen MR colonography versus conventional colonoscopy. Radiology. 2006;238:143–9.

19. Quo JH, Teng GJ, Zhu GY, He SC, Deng G, He J. Self-expandable stent loaded with 1251 seeds: feasibility and safety in a rabbit model. Eur J Radiol. 2007;61:356–61.

20. Kim JH, Song HY, Shin JH et al. Metallic stent placement in the palliative treatment of malignant gastroduodenal obstructions: prospective evaluation of results and factors influencing outcome in 213 patients. Gastrointest Endosc. 2007;66:256–64.

21. He GJ, Gao QY, Xu SH et al. 103Pd radioactive stent inhibits biliary duct restenosis and reduces smooth muscle actin expression during duct healing in dogs. Hepatobil Pancreat Dis Int. 2006;5:595–8.

22. Meng B, Wang J, Zhu N, Meng QY, Cui FZ, Xu YX. Study of biodegradable and self-expandable PLLA helical biliary stent *in vivo* and *in vitro*. J Mater Sci Mater Med. 2006:17:611–17.

23. Han J, Shin JH, Lee SS et al. Influence of a paclitaxel-eluting covered metallic stent on tissue hyperplasia: an experimental study in a canine biliary model. Gastrointest Endosc. 2007;65:AB219.

24. Lee DK, Suk KT, Kim JW et al. A clinical trial of a metallic stent covered with a paclitaxel-incorporated membrane for patients with malignant biliary obstruction. Gastrointest Endosc. 2007;65:AB235.

25. Park PO, Bergstrom M, Ikeda K et al. Endoscopic pyloroplasty with full-thickness transgastric and transduodenal myotomy with sutured closure. Gastrointest Endosc. 2007;66:116–20.

26. Pasricha PJ, Hawari R, Ahmed I et al. Submucosal endoscopic esophageal myotomy: a novel experimental approach for the treatment of achalasia. Endoscopy. 2007;39:761–4.

27. Fritscher-Ravens A, Mosse CA, Mukherjee D, Mills T, Park PO, Swain CP. Transluminal endosurgery: single lumen access anastomotic device for flexible endoscopy. Gastrointest Endosc. 2003;58:585–91.
28. Fritscher-Ravens A, Mosse CA, Ikeda K, Swain P. Endoscopic transgastric lymphadenectomy by using EUS for selection and guidance. Gastrointest Endosc. 2006;63:302–6.
29. Fritscher-Ravens A, Ganbari A, Mosse CA, Swain P, Koehler P, Patel K. Transesophageal endoscopic ultrasound-guided access to the heart. Endoscopy. 2007;39:385–9.
30. Thompson CC, Ryou M, Rothstein Rl et al. Stomach – direct drive endoscopic system for endoluminal and NOTES applications. The DAVE Project, from http://dave1.mgh. harvard.edu/ViewRlms.cfm?filmjd=8l2.

12
State-of-the-Art Lecture: Natural orifice transluminal endoscopic surgery (NOTES)

B. DALLEMAGNE

INTRODUCTION

A few years back, endoscopists improved the range of flexible endoscopes by implementing therapeutic capabilities (interventional endoscopy) to the diagnostic ones that they had had since the beginning of the twentieth century.

During the 1980s endoscopes were fitted with cameras. This allowed one to view on a screen the work in progress, and led to a boost in endoscopic surgery.

Endoscopes were first applied for the resection of polyps and sphincterotomies, followed recently by superficial tumour resections at all levels of the digestive tube accessible via natural orifices.

The majority of interventional gastroenterologists had as a major worry the complications induced by perforation of the visceral wall, since any opening to the peritoneal cavity could potentially cause infection, abscess, peritonitis, or fistula.

Percutaneous endoscopic gastrostomy was the first surgical endoscopic technique that intentionally perforated a hollow organ[1]. Following this, transluminal drainage of post-pancreatitis collections progressively accustomed some endoscopists to an extraluminal approach[2]. The surgeon's moves were limited to drainage of fluid collections and abscesses. The first to have used a surgical endoscopic technique for the resection of an organ's segment, and as such an opening to the peritoneal cavity, is G. Buess, who described in 1984 transanal endoscopic surgery[3]. Complete resections of low sigmoid or rectal tumours with parietal defect suturing are performed through an adapted rectoscope using specific instrumentation.

These different applications probably spurred the gastroenterologists' imagination assembled in the Apollo group. This group, formed by American and Chinese university physicians, aimed at enlarging the scope of application of endoscopic surgery. One of its members, A. Kalloo, unveiled the concept of transgastric surgery in 2000, in an abstract submitted to the *Digestive Disease Week* (DDW). This presentation was followed in 2004 by a publication in

GastroIntestinal Endoscopy in which the authors reported a survival study following hepatic biopsies performed via a transgastric endoscopic route. The stomach's wall incision was closed by endoscopic clips. No complication was observed during the survival follow-up of 14 days[4]. This article sparked enthusiasm in the medical community but also in the surgical community. In 2005 the ASGE and the SAGES created a work group aiming at studying all the parameters linked to this new approach to the peritoneal cavity. The group published a white paper listing all the potential constraints, as well as the technical and physiological problems, that need to be studied before a clinical application of natural orifice transluminal endoscopic surgery (NOTES)[5].

THE CONCEPT

The work group created by the ASGE and the SAGES was called the Natural Orifice Surgery Consortium for Assessment and Research (NOSCAR), a name that perfectly embodies the NOTES concept. The aim of scarless surgery is to rule out the complications related to abdominal wall incisions (risks of infection, eventration), to reduce the intraoperative and postoperative pain whilst providing cosmetic and possible psychological benefits to patients. The objective is to enhance the benefits already attributed to laparoscopic surgery over conventional surgery.

If the concept was initially based on the use of a transgastric route, this one rapidly revealed some difficulties specifically related to the exposure and dissection of the operative field in positions technically unfavourable (e.g. retroflexion), and impaired by the limited range of technologies currently available for the closure of gastric incisions[5].

Such difficulties prompted the work groups to envisage and study other approaches, and opt for other natural orifices (vagina, rectum, colon, and bladder).

Numerous animal model experimentations have been reported, some with survival studies, amply covering the scope of standard interventions such as cholecystectomies, splenectomies, appendicectomies, adnexectomies, hysterectomies, pancreatectomies, and nephrectomies[6–14]. The modalities for closure of transluminal accesses are subject to intensive laboratory research studies. Between 2004 and 2007 the IRCAD–EITS team performed more than 300 experimental studies in the field in parallel to developing surgical applications. The results obtained in the survival studies were very encouraging. The technologies studied must still be improved before any clinical application[15–18] is possible.

Other studies focus on the consequences of opening a hollow organ within the peritoneal cavity with the risks of infection, adhesions, and response to intraoperative stress. Generally speaking, these studies prove that this novel approach has physiological consequences similar to those in laparoscopic surgery[19,20]. The benefits related to the absence of incision and scar will only be assessed in the clinical series that began in 2007 in the frame of stringent protocols.

THE CLINICAL APPLICATION

The clinical assessment of the NOTES concept, *no scar*, must ideally avoid the pitfalls and potential complications related to the incision of a hollow organ in the peritoneal cavity. Additionally, it must take into account the current technological limitations of endoscopes and surgical instruments.

It is within this constraining framework that IRCAD–EITS has rapidly geared up its research studies towards the use of the transvaginal route. This approach, that has been used for ages by gynaecologists, provides extremely low complication rates (infection: 0.001%, bleeding: 0.002%)[21]. Following an intense experimental programme the first NOTES cholecystectomy was performed in April 2007[22]. This marked a watershed in surgical history which has made it possible to confirm the current-day technological constraints and the hybrid approach (with a further laparoscopic port used for clip application and specific steps of dissection) is presently used.

Other surgical teams have also opted for this hybrid solution, by using one or two additional ports[23].

The application of transgastric cholecystectomy was undertaken within strict ethical protocols given the unknown related to the closure of the abdominal wall. The teams at work, among which are the one at IRCAD–EITS, have also favoured a hybrid approach that ensures safe closure of the gastric wall using sutures.

The immediate results of either approach are satisfying, with a decrease in postoperative pain when compared to laparoscopy. However, it must be noted that the clinical series are very scarce and that no conclusions can be currently drawn.

THE FUTURE

The future of NOTES is fundamentally related to the development of technologies which must allow the surgeon to correctly visualize the anatomical structures in order to expose, retract, divide, and suture them[24]. It is a huge challenge to take up; therefore research and development agencies are calling for the skills of surgeons, endoscopists, robotic and IT engineers.

If the concept proves its rationale, it will most probably bring about a profound change in the surgical environment and the ways in which surgeons practise and interact.

References

1. Gauderer MW, Ponsky JL, Izant RJ Jr. Gastrostomy without laparotomy: a percutaneous endoscopic technique. J Pediatr Surg. 1980;15:872–5.
2. Kozarek RA, Brayko CM, Harlan J, Sanowski RA, Cintora I, Kovac A. Endoscopic drainage of pancreatic pseudocysts. Gastrointest Endosc. 1985;31:322–7.
3. Buess G, Hutterer F, Theiss J, Bobel M, Isselhard W, Pichlmaier H. [A system for a transanal endoscopic rectum operation]. Chirurg. 1984;55:677–80.
4. Kalloo AN, Singh VK, Jagannath SB et al. Flexible transgastric peritoneoscopy: a novel approach to diagnostic and therapeutic interventions in the peritoneal cavity. Gastrointest Endosc. 2004;60:114–17.

5. ASGE/SAGES Working Group on Natural Orifice Translumenal Endoscopic Surgery White Paper, October 2005. Gastrointest Endosc. 2006;63:199–203.

6. Jagannath SB, Kantsevoy SV, Vaughn CA et al. Peroral transgastric endoscopic ligation of fallopian tubes with long-term survival in a porcine model. Gastrointest Endosc. 2005;61:449–53.

7. Kantsevoy SV, Jagannath SB, Niiyama H et al. Endoscopic gastrojejunostomy with survival in a porcine model. Gastrointest Endosc. 2005;62:287–92.

8. Park PO, Bergstrom M, Ikeda K, Fritscher-Ravens A, Swain P. Experimental studies of transgastric gallbladder surgery: cholecystectomy and cholecystogastric anastomosis (videos). Gastrointest Endosc. 2005;61:601–6.

9. Kantsevoy SV, Hu B, Jagannath SB et al. Transgastric endoscopic splenectomy: is it possible? Surg Endosc. 2006; 20:522–5.

10. Lima E, Rolanda C, Pego JM et al. Transvesical endoscopic peritoneoscopy: a novel 5 mm port for intra-abdominal scarless surgery. J Urol. 2006;176:802–5.

11. Pai RD, Fong DG, Bundga ME, Odze RD, Rattner DW, Thompson CC. Transcolonic endoscopic cholecystectomy: a NOTES survival study in a porcine model (with video). Gastrointest Endosc. 2006;64:428–34.

12. Sumiyama K, Gostout CJ, Rajan E et al. Pilot study of the porcine uterine horn as an in vivo appendicitis model for development of endoscopic transgastric appendectomy. Gastrointest Endosc. 2006;64:808–12.

13. Branco AW, Filho AJ, Kondo W et al. Hybrid transvaginal nephrectomy. Eur Urol. 2008;53:1290–4.

14. Perretta S, Dallemagne B, Coumaros D, Marescaux J. Natural orifice transluminal endoscopic surgery: transgastric cholecystectomy in a survival porcine model. Surg Endosc. 2008;22:1126–30.

15. Sclabas GM, Swain P, Swanstrom LL. Endoluminal methods for gastrotomy closure in natural orifice transenteric surgery (NOTES). Surg Innov. 2006;13:23–30.

16. Cios TJ, Reavis KM, Renton DR et al. Gastrotomy closure using bioabsorbable plugs in a canine model. Surg Endosc. 2008;22:961–6.

17. McGee MF, Marks JM, Jin J et al. Complete endoscopic closure of gastric defects using a full-thickness tissue plicating device. J Gastrointest Surg. 2008;12:38–45.

18. Perretta S, Sereno S, Forgione A et al. A new method to close the gastrotomy by using a cardiac septal occluder: long-term survival study in a porcine model. Gastrointest Endosc. 2007;66:809–13.

19. Meireles O, Kantsevoy SV, Kalloo AN et al. Comparison of intraabdominal pressures using the gastroscope and laparoscope for transgastric surgery. Surg Endosc. 2007;21:998–1001.

20. von Delius S, Huber W, Feussner H et al. Effect of pneumoperitoneum on hemodynamics and inspiratory pressures during natural orifice transluminal endoscopic surgery (NOTES): an experimental, controlled study in an acute porcine model. Endoscopy. 2007;39:854–61.

21. Watrelot A. Place of transvaginal fertiloscopy in the management of tubal factor disease. Reprod Biomed Online. 2007;15:389–95.

22. Marescaux J, Dallemagne B, Perretta S, Wattiez A, Mutter D, Coumaros D. Surgery without scars: report of transluminal cholecystectomy in a human being. Arch Surg. 2007;142:823–6.

23. Zorron R, Maggioni LC, Pombo L, Oliveira AL, Carvalho GL, Filgueiras M. NOTES transvaginal cholecystectomy: preliminary clinical application. Surg Endosc. 2008;22:542–7.

24. Swanstrom LL, Whiteford M, Khajanchee Y. Developing essential tools to enable transgastric surgery. Surg Endosc. 2008;22:600–4.

Index

Falk Symposium Series

43. Reutter W, Popper H, Arias IM, Heinrich PC, Keppler D, Landmann L, eds.: *Modulation of Liver Cell Expression*. Falk Symposium No. 43. 1987
ISBN: 0-85200-677-2*
44. Boyer JL, Bianchi L, eds.: *Liver Cirrhosis*. Falk Symposium No. 44. 1987
ISBN: 0-85200-993-3*
45. Paumgartner G, Stiehl A, Gerok W, eds.: *Bile Acids and the Liver*. Falk Symposium No. 45. 1987
ISBN: 0-85200-675-6*
46. Goebell H, Peskar BM, Malchow H, eds.: *Inflammatory Bowel Diseases – Basic Research & Clinical Implications*. Falk Symposium No. 46. 1988
ISBN: 0-7462-0067-6*
47. Bianchi L, Holt P, James OFW, Butler RN, eds.: *Aging in Liver and Gastrointestinal Tract*. Falk Symposium No. 47. 1988   ISBN: 0-7462-0066-8*
48. Heilmann C, ed.: *Calcium-Dependent Processes in the Liver*. Falk Symposium No. 48. 1988   ISBN: 0-7462-0075-7*
50. Singer MV, Goebell H, eds.: *Nerves and the Gastrointestinal Tract*. Falk Symposium No. 50. 1989   ISBN: 0-7462-0114-1
51. Bannasch P, Keppler D, Weber G, eds.: *Liver Cell Carcinoma*. Falk Symposium No. 51. 1989   ISBN: 0-7462-0111-7
52. Paumgartner G, Stiehl A, Gerok W, eds.: *Trends in Bile Acid Research*. Falk Symposium No. 52. 1989   ISBN: 0-7462-0112-5
53. Paumgartner G, Stiehl A, Barbara L, Roda E, eds.: *Strategies for the Treatment of Hepatobiliary Diseases*. Falk Symposium No. 53. 1990   ISBN: 0-7923-8903-4
54. Bianchi L, Gerok W, Maier K-P, Deinhardt F, eds.: *Infectious Diseases of the Liver*. Falk Symposium No. 54. 1990   ISBN: 0-7923-8902-6
55. Falk Symposium No. 55 not published
55B. Hadziselimovic F, Herzog B, Bürgin-Wolff A, eds.: *Inflammatory Bowel Disease and Coeliac Disease in Children*. International Falk Symposium. 1990
ISBN 0-7462-0125-7
56. Williams CN, eds.: *Trends in Inflammatory Bowel Disease Therapy*. Falk Symposium No. 56. 1990   ISBN: 0-7923-8952-2
57. Bock KW, Gerok W, Matern S, Schmid R, eds.: *Hepatic Metabolism and Disposition of Endo- and Xenobiotics*. Falk Symposium No. 57. 1991   ISBN: 0-7923-8953-0
58. Paumgartner G, Stiehl A, Gerok W, eds.: *Bile Acids as Therapeutic Agents: From Basic Science to Clinical Practice*. Falk Symposium No. 58. 1991   ISBN: 0-7923-8954-9
59. Halter F, Garner A, Tytgat GNJ, eds.: *Mechanisms of Peptic Ulcer Healing*. Falk Symposium No. 59. 1991   ISBN: 0-7923-8955-7
60. Goebell H, Ewe K, Malchow H, Koelbel Ch, eds.: *Inflammatory Bowel Diseases – Progress in Basic Research and Clinical Implications*. Falk Symposium No. 60. 1991
ISBN: 0-7923-8956-5
61. Falk Symposium No. 61 not published
62. Dowling RH, Folsch UR, Löser Ch, eds.: *Polyamines in the Gastrointestinal Tract*. Falk Symposium No. 62. 1992   ISBN: 0-7923-8976-X
63. Lentze MJ, Reichen J, eds.: *Paediatric Cholestasis: Novel Approaches to Treatment*. Falk Symposium No. 63. 1992   ISBN: 0-7923-8977-8
64. Demling L, Frühmorgen P, eds.: *Non-Neoplastic Diseases of the Anorectum*. Falk Symposium No. 64. 1992   ISBN: 0-7923-8979-4
64B. Gressner AM, Ramadori G, eds.: *Molecular and Cell Biology of Liver Fibrogenesis*. International Falk Symposium. 1992   ISBN: 0-7923-8980-8

*These titles were published under the MTP Press imprint.

Falk Symposium Series

65. Hadziselimovic F, Herzog B, eds.: *Inflammatory Bowel Diseases and Morbus Hirschprung*. Falk Symposium No. 65. 1992   ISBN: 0-7923-8995-6

66. Martin F, McLeod RS, Sutherland LR, Williams CN, eds.: *Trends in Inflammatory Bowel Disease Therapy*. Falk Symposium No. 66. 1993   ISBN: 0-7923-8827-5

67. Schölmerich J, Kruis W, Goebell H, Hohenberger W, Gross V, eds.: *Inflammatory Bowel Diseases – Pathophysiology as Basis of Treatment*. Falk Symposium No. 67. 1993   ISBN: 0-7923-8996-4

68. Paumgartner G, Stiehl A, Gerok W, eds.: *Bile Acids and The Hepatobiliary System: From Basic Science to Clinical Practice*. Falk Symposium No. 68. 1993   ISBN: 0-7923-8829-1

69. Schmid R, Bianchi L, Gerok W, Maier K-P, eds.: *Extrahepatic Manifestations in Liver Diseases*. Falk Symposium No. 69. 1993   ISBN: 0-7923-8821-6

70. Meyer zum Büschenfelde K-H, Hoofnagle J, Manns M, eds.: *Immunology and Liver*. Falk Symposium No. 70. 1993   ISBN: 0-7923-8830-5

71. Surrenti C, Casini A, Milani S, Pinzani M , eds.: *Fat-Storing Cells and Liver Fibrosis*. Falk Symposium No. 71. 1994   ISBN: 0-7923-8842-9

72. Rachmilewitz D, ed.: *Inflammatory Bowel Diseases – 1994*. Falk Symposium No. 72. 1994   ISBN: 0-7923-8845-3

73. Binder HJ, Cummings J, Soergel KH, eds.: *Short Chain Fatty Acids*. Falk Symposium No. 73. 1994   ISBN: 0-7923-8849-6

73B. Möllmann HW, May B, eds.: *Glucocorticoid Therapy in Chronic Inflammatory Bowel Disease: from basic principles to rational therapy*. International Falk Workshop. 1996   ISBN 0-7923-8708-2

74. Keppler D, Jungermann K, eds.: *Transport in the Liver*. Falk Symposium No. 74. 1994   ISBN: 0-7923-8858-5

74B. Stange EF, ed.: *Chronic Inflammatory Bowel Disease*. Falk Symposium. 1995   ISBN: 0-7923-8876-3

75. van Berge Henegouwen GP, van Hoek B, De Groote J, Matern S, Stockbrügger RW, eds.: *Cholestatic Liver Diseases: New Strategies for Prevention and Treatment of Hepatobiliary and Cholestatic Liver Diseases*. Falk Symposium 75. 1994.   ISBN: 0-7923-8867-4

76. Monteiro E, Tavarela Veloso F, eds.: *Inflammatory Bowel Diseases: New Insights into Mechanisms of Inflammation and Challenges in Diagnosis and Treatment*. Falk Symposium 76. 1995.   ISBN 0-7923-8884-4

77. Singer MV, Ziegler R, Rohr G, eds.: *Gastrointestinal Tract and Endocrine System*. Falk Symposium 77. 1995.   ISBN 0-7923-8877-1

78. Decker K, Gerok W, Andus T, Gross V, eds.: *Cytokines and the Liver*. Falk Symposium 78. 1995.   ISBN 0-7923-8878-X

79. Holstege A, Schölmerich J, Hahn EG, eds.: *Portal Hypertension*. Falk Symposium 79. 1995.   ISBN 0-7923-8879-8

80. Hofmann AF, Paumgartner G, Stiehl A, eds.: *Bile Acids in Gastroenterology: Basic and Clinical Aspects*. Falk Symposium 80. 1995   ISBN 0-7923-8880-1

81. Riecken EO, Stallmach A, Zeitz M, Heise W, eds.: *Malignancy and Chronic Inflammation in the Gastrointestinal Tract – New Concepts*. Falk Symposium 81. 1995 ISBN 0-7923-8889-5

82. Fleig WE, ed.: *Inflammatory Bowel Diseases: New Developments and Standards*. Falk Symposium 82. 1995   ISBN 0-7923-8890-6

82B. Paumgartner G, Beuers U, eds.: *Bile Acids in Liver Diseases*. International Falk Workshop. 1995   ISBN 0-7923-8891-7

Falk Symposium Series

83. Dobrilla G, Felder M, de Pretis G, eds.: *Advances in Hepatobiliary and Pancreatic Diseases: Special Clinical Topics.* Falk Symposium 83. 1995.   ISBN 0-7923-8892-5
84. Fromm H, Leuschner U, eds.: *Bile Acids – Cholestasis – Gallstones: Advances in Basic and Clinical Bile Acid Research.* Falk Symposium 84. 1995   ISBN 0-7923-8893-3
85. Tytgat GNJ, Bartelsman JFWM, van Deventer SJH, eds.: *Inflammatory Bowel Diseases.* Falk Symposium 85. 1995   ISBN 0-7923-8894-1
86. Berg PA, Leuschner U, eds.: *Bile Acids and Immunology.* Falk Symposium 86. 1996
     ISBN 0-7923-8700-7
87. Schmid R, Bianchi L, Blum HE, Gerok W, Maier KP, Stalder GA, eds.: *Acute and Chronic Liver Diseases: Molecular Biology and Clinics.* Falk Symposium 87. 1996
     ISBN 0-7923-8701-5
88. Blum HE, Wu GY, Wu CH, eds.: *Molecular Diagnosis and Gene Therapy.* Falk Symposium 88. 1996   ISBN 0-7923-8702-3
88B. Poupon RE, Reichen J, eds.: *Surrogate Markers to Assess Efficacy of TReatment in Chronic Liver Diseases.* International Falk Workshop. 1996   ISBN 0-7923-8705-8
89. Reyes HB, Leuschner U, Arias IM, eds.: *Pregnancy, Sex Hormones and the Liver.* Falk Symposium 89. 1996   ISBN 0-7923-8704-X
89B. Broelsch CE, Burdelski M, Rogiers X, eds.: *Cholestatic Liver Diseases in Children and Adults.* International Falk Workshop. 1996   ISBN 0-7923-8710-4
90. Lam S-K, Paumgartner P, Wang B, eds.: *Update on Hepatobiliary Diseases 1996.* Falk Symposium 90. 1996   ISBN 0-7923-8715-5
91. Hadziselimovic F, Herzog B, eds.: *Inflammatory Bowel Diseases and Chronic Recurrent Abdominal Pain.* Falk Symposium 91. 1996   ISBN 0-7923-8722-8
91B. Alvaro D, Benedetti A, Strazzabosco M, eds.: *Vanishing Bile Duct Syndrome – Pathophysiology and Treatment.* International Falk Workshop. 1996
     ISBN 0-7923-8721-X
92. Gerok W, Loginov AS, Pokrowskij VI, eds.: *New Trends in Hepatology 1996.* Falk Symposium 92. 1997   ISBN 0-7923-8723-6
93. Paumgartner G, Stiehl A, Gerok W, eds.: *Bile Acids in Hepatobiliary Diseases – Basic Research and Clinical Application.* Falk Symposium 93. 1997   ISBN 0-7923-8725-2
94. Halter F, Winton D, Wright NA, eds.: *The Gut as a Model in Cell and Molecular Biology.* Falk Symposium 94. 1997   ISBN 0-7923-8726-0
94B. Kruse-Jarres JD, Schölmerich J, eds.: *Zinc and Diseases of the Digestive Tract.* International Falk Workshop. 1997   ISBN 0-7923-8724-4
95. Ewe K, Eckardt VF, Enck P, eds.: *Constipation and Anorectal Insufficiency.* Falk Symposium 95. 1997   ISBN 0-7923-8727-9
96. Andus T, Goebell H, Layer P, Schölmerich J, eds.: *Inflammatory Bowel Disease – from Bench to Bedside.* Falk Symposium 96. 1997   ISBN 0-7923-8728-7
97. Campieri M, Bianchi-Porro G, Fiocchi C, Schölmerich J, eds. *Clinical Challenges in Inflammatory Bowel Diseases: Diagnosis, Prognosis and Treatment.* Falk Symposium 97. 1998   ISBN 0-7923-8733-3
98. Lembcke B, Kruis W, Sartor RB, eds. *Systemic Manifestations of IBD: The Pending Challenge for Subtle Diagnosis and Treatment.* Falk Symposium 98. 1998
     ISBN 0-7923-8734-1
99. Goebell H, Holtmann G, Talley NJ, eds. *Functional Dyspepsia and Irritable Bowel Syndrome: Concepts and Controversies.* Falk Symposium 99. 1998
     ISBN 0-7923-8735-X
100. Blum HE, Bode Ch, Bode JCh, Sartor RB, eds. *Gut and the Liver.* Falk Symposium 100. 1998   ISBN 0-7923-8736-8

Falk Symposium Series

101. Rachmilewitz D, ed. *V International Symposium on Inflammatory Bowel Diseases.* Falk Symposium 101. 1998   ISBN 0-7923-8743-0
102. Manns MP, Boyer JL, Jansen PLM, Reichen J, eds. *Cholestatic Liver Diseases.* Falk Symposium 102. 1998   ISBN 0-7923-8746-5
102B. Manns MP, Chapman RW, Stiehl A, Wiesner R, eds. *Primary Sclerosing Cholangitis.* International Falk Workshop. 1998.   ISBN 0-7923-8745-7
103. Häussinger D, Jungermann K, eds. *Liver and Nervous System.* Falk Symposium 102. 1998   ISBN 0-7924-8742-2
103B. Häussinger D, Heinrich PC, eds. *Signalling in the Liver.* International Falk Workshop. 1998   ISBN 0-7923-8744-9
103C. Fleig W, ed. *Normal and Malignant Liver Cell Growth.* International Falk Workshop. 1998   ISBN 0-7923-8748-1
104. Stallmach A, Zeitz M, Strober W, MacDonald TT, Lochs H, eds. *Induction and Modulation of Gastrointestinal Inflammation.* Falk Symposium 104. 1998
ISBN 0-7923-8747-3
105. Emmrich J, Liebe S, Stange EF, eds. *Innovative Concepts in Inflammatory Bowel Diseases.* Falk Symposium 105. 1999   ISBN 0-7923-8749-X
106. Rutgeerts P, Colombel J-F, Hanauer SB, Schölmerich J, Tytgat GNJ, van Gossum A, eds. *Advances in Inflammatory Bowel Diseases.* Falk Symposium 106. 1999
ISBN 0-7923-8750-3
107. Špičák J, Boyer J, Gilat T, Kotrlik K, Mareček Z, Paumgartner G, eds. *Diseases of the Liver and the Bile Ducts – New Aspects and Clinical Implications.* Falk Symposium 107. 1999   ISBN 0-7923-8751-1
108. Paumgartner G, Stiehl A, Gerok W, Keppler D, Leuschner U, eds. *Bile Acids and Cholestasis.* Falk Symposium 108. 1999   ISBN 0-7923-8752-X
109. Schmiegel W, Schölmerich J, eds. *Colorectal Cancer – Molecular Mechanisms, Premalignant State and its Prevention.* Falk Symposium 109. 1999
ISBN 0-7923-8753-8
110. Domschke W, Stoll R, Brasitus TA, Kagnoff MF, eds. *Intestinal Mucosa and its Diseases – Pathophysiology and Clinics.* Falk Symposium 110. 1999
ISBN 0-7923-8754-6
110B. Northfield TC, Ahmed HA, Jazwari RP, Zentler-Munro PL, eds. *Bile Acids in Hepatobiliary Disease.* Falk Workshop. 2000   ISBN 0-7923-8755-4
111. Rogler G, Kullmann F, Rutgeerts P, Sartor RB, Schölmerich J, eds. *IBD at the End of its First Century.* Falk Symposium 111. 2000   ISBN 0-7923-8756-2
112. Krammer HJ, Singer MV, eds. *Neurogastroenterology: From the Basics to the Clinics.* Falk Symposium 112. 2000   ISBN 0-7923-8757-0
113. Andus T, Rogler G, Schlottmann K, Frick E, Adler G, Schmiegel W, Zeitz M, Schölmerich J, eds. *Cytokines and Cell Homeostasis in the Gastrointestinal Tract.* Falk Symposium 113. 2000   ISBN 0-7923-8758-9
114. Manns MP, Paumgartner G, Leuschner U, eds. *Immunology and Liver.* Falk Symposium 114. 2000   ISBN 0-7923-8759-7
115. Boyer JL, Blum HE, Maier K-P, Sauerbruch T, Stalder GA, eds. *Liver Cirrhosis and its Development.* Falk Symposium 115. 2000   ISBN 0-7923-8760-0
116. Riemann JF, Neuhaus H, eds. *Interventional Endoscopy in Hepatology.* Falk Symposium 116. 2000   ISBN 0-7923-8761-9
116A. Dienes HP, Schirmacher P, Brechot C, Okuda K, eds. *Chronic Hepatitis: New Concepts of Pathogenesis, Diagnosis and Treatment.* Falk Workshop. 2000
ISBN 0-7923-8763-5

Falk Symposium Series

117. Gerbes AL, Beuers U, Jüngst D, Pape GR, Sackmann M, Sauerbruch T, eds. *Hepatology 2000 – Symposium in Honour of Gustav Paumgartner.* Falk Symposium 117. 2000 ISBN 0-7923-8765-1

117A. Acalovschi M, Paumgartner G, eds. *Hepatobiliary Diseases: Cholestasis and Gallstones.* Falk Workshop. 2000 ISBN 0-7923-8770-8

118. Frühmorgen P, Bruch H-P, eds. *Non-Neoplastic Diseases of the Anorectum.* Falk Symposium 118. 2001 ISBN 0-7923-8766-X

119. Fellermann K, Jewell DP, Sandborn WJ, Schölmerich J, Stange EF, eds. *Immunosuppression in Inflammatory Bowel Diseases – Standards, New Developments, Future Trends.* Falk Symposium 119. 2001 ISBN 0-7923-8767-8

120. van Berge Henegouwen GP, Keppler D, Leuschner U, Paumgartner G, Stiehl A, eds. *Biology of Bile Acids in Health and Disease.* Falk Symposium 120. 2001 ISBN 0-7923-8768-6

121. Leuschner U, James OFW, Dancygier H, eds. *Steatohepatitis (NASH and ASH).* Falk Symposium 121. 2001 ISBN 0-7923-8769-4

121A. Matern S, Boyer JL, Keppler D, Meier-Abt PJ, eds. *Hepatobiliary Transport: From Bench to Bedside.* Falk Workshop. 2001 ISBN 0-7923-8771-6

122. Campieri M, Fiocchi C, Hanauer SB, Jewell DP, Rachmilewitz R, Schölmerich J, eds. *Inflammatory Bowel Disease – A Clinical Case Approach to Pathophysiology, Diagnosis, and Treatment.* Falk Symposium 122. 2002 ISBN 0-7923-8772-4

123. Rachmilewitz D, Modigliani R, Podolsky DK, Sachar DB, Tozun N, eds. *VI International Symposium on Inflammatory Bowel Diseases.* Falk Symposium 123. 2002 ISBN 0-7923-8773-2

124. Hagenmüller F, Manns MP, Musmann H-G, Riemann JF, eds. *Medical Imaging in Gastroenterology and Hepatology.* Falk Symposium 124. 2002 ISBN 0-7923-8774-0

125. Gressner AM, Heinrich PC, Matern S, eds. *Cytokines in Liver Injury and Repair.* Falk Symposium 125. 2002 ISBN 0-7923-8775-9

126. Gupta S, Jansen PLM, Klempnauer J, Manns MP, eds. *Hepatocyte Transplantation.* Falk Symposium 126. 2002 ISBN 0-7923-8776-7

127. Hadziselimovic F, ed. *Autoimmune Diseases in Paediatric Gastroenterology.* Falk Symposium 127. 2002 ISBN 0-7923-8778-3

127A. Berr F, Bruix J, Hauss J, Wands J, Wittekind Ch, eds. *Malignant Liver Tumours: Basic Concepts and Clinical Management.* Falk Workshop. 2002 ISBN 0-7923-8779-1

128. Scheppach W, Scheurlen M, eds. *Exogenous Factors in Colonic Carcinogenesis.* Falk Symposium 128. 2002 ISBN 0-7923-8780-5

129. Paumgartner G, Keppler D, Leuschner U, Stiehl A, eds. *Bile Acids: From Genomics to Disease and Therapy.* Falk Symposium 129. 2002 ISBN 0-7923-8781-3

129A. Leuschner U, Berg PA, Holtmeier J, eds. *Bile Acids and Pregnancy.* Falk Workshop. 2002 ISBN 0-7923-8782-1

130. Holtmann G, Talley NJ, eds. *Gastrointestinal Inflammation and Disturbed Gut Function: The Challenge of New Concepts.* Falk Symposium 130. 2003 ISBN 0-7923-8783-X

131. Herfarth H, Feagan BJ, Folsch UR, Schölmerich J, Vatn MH, Zeitz M, eds. *Targets of Treatment in Chronic Inflammatory Bowel Diseases.* Falk Symposium 131. 2003 ISBN 0-7923-8784-8

132. Galle PR, Gerken G, Schmidt WE, Wiedenmann B, eds. *Disease Progression and Carcinogenesis in the Gastrointestinal Tract.* Falk Symposium 132. 2003 ISBN 0-7923-8785-6

Falk Symposium Series

132A. Staritz M, Adler G, Knuth A, Schmiegel W, Schmoll H-J, eds. *Side-effects of Chemotherapy on the Gastrointestinal Tract*. Falk Workshop. 2003
ISBN 0-7923-8791-0

132B. Reutter W, Schuppan D, Tauber R, Zeitz M, eds. *Cell Adhesion Molecules in Health and Disease*. Falk Workshop. 2003   ISBN 0-7923-8786-4

133. Duchmann R, Blumberg R, Neurath M, Schölmerich J, Strober W, Zeitz M. *Mechanisms of Intestinal Inflammation: Implications for Therapeutic Intervention in IBD*. Falk Symposium 133. 2004   ISBN 0-7923-8787-2

134. Dignass A, Lochs H, Stange E. *Trends and Controversies in IBD – Evidence-Based Approach or Individual Management?* Falk Symposium 134. 2004
ISBN 0-7923-8788-0

134A. Dignass A, Gross HJ, Buhr V, James OFW. *Topical Steroids in Gastroenterology and Hepatology*. Falk Workshop. 2004   ISBN 0-7923-8789-9

135. Lukáš M, Manns MP, Špičák J, Stange EF, eds. *Immunological Diseases of Liver and Gut*. Falk Symposium 135. 2004   ISBN 0-7923-8792-9

136. Leuschner U, Broomé U, Stiehl A, eds. *Cholestatic Liver Diseases: Therapeutic Options and Perspectives*. Falk Symposium 136. 2004   ISBN 0-7923-8793-7

137. Blum HE, Maier KP, Rodés J, Sauerbruch T, eds. *Liver Diseases: Advances in Treatment and Prevention*. Falk Symposium 137. 2004   ISBN 0-7923-8794-5

138. Blum HE, Manns MP, eds. *State of the Art of Hepatology: Molecular and Cell Biology*. Falk Symposium 138. 2004   ISBN 0-7923-8795-3

138A. Hayashi N, Manns MP, eds. *Prevention of Progression in Chronic Liver Disease: An Update on SNMC (Stronger Neo-Minophagen C)*. Falk Workshop. 2004
ISBN 0-7923-8796-1

139. Adler G, Blum HE, Fuchs M, Stange EF, eds. *Gallstones: Pathogenesis and Treatment*. Falk Symposium 139. 2004   ISBN 0-7923-8798-8

140. Colombel J-F, Gasché C, Schölmerich J, Vucelic C, eds. *Inflammatory Bowel Disease: Translation from Basic Research to Clinical Practice*. Falk Symposium 140. 2005.   ISBN 1-4020-2847-4

141. Paumgartner G, Keppler D, Leuschner U, Stiehl A, eds. *Bile Acid Biology and its Therapeutic Implications*. Falk Symposium 141. 2005   ISBN 1-4020-2893-8

142. Dienes H-P, Leuschner U, Lohse AW, Manns MP, eds. *Autoimmune Liver Disease*. Falk Symposium 142. 2005   ISBN 1-4020-2894-6

143. Ammann RW, Büchler MW, Adler G, DiMagno EP, Sarner M, eds. *Pancreatitis: Advances in Pathobiology, Diagnosis and Treatment*. Falk Symposium 143. 2005
ISBN 1-4020-2895-4

144. Adler G, Blum AL, Blum HE, Leuschner U, Manns MP, Mössner J, Sartor RB, Schölmerich J, eds. *Gastroenterology Yesterday – Today – Tomorrow: A Review and Preview*. Falk Symposium 144. 2005   ISBN 1-4020-2896-2

145. Henne-Bruns D, Buttenschön K, Fuchs M, Lohse AW, eds. *Artificial Liver Support*. Falk Symposium 145. 2005   ISBN 1-4020-3239-0

146. Blumberg RS, Gangl A, Manns MP, Tilg H, Zeitz M, eds. *Gut–Liver Interactions: Basic and Clinical Concepts*. Falk Symposium 146. 2005   ISBN 1-4020-4143-8

147. Jewell DP, Colombel JF, Peña AS, Tromm A, Warren BS, eds. *Colitis: Diagnosis and Therapeutic Strategies*. Falk Symposium 147. 2006   ISBN 1-4020-4315-5

148. Kruis W, Forbes A, Jauch K-W, Kreis ME, Wexner SD, eds. *Diverticular Disease: Emerging Evidence in a Common Condition*. Falk Symposium 148. 2006
ISBN 1-4020- 4317-1

149. van Cutsem E, Rustgi AK, Schmiegel W, Zeitz M, eds. *Highlights in Gastrointestinal Oncology*. Falk Symposium 149. 2006.   ISBN 1-4020-5108-5

Falk Symposium Series

150. Galle PR, Gerken G, Schmidt WE, Wiedenmann B, eds. *Disease Progression and Disease Prevention in Hepatology and Gastroenterology.* Falk Symposium 150. 2006
ISBN 1-4020-5109-3

151. Fraser A, Gibson PR, Hibi T, Qian J-M, Schölmerich, eds. *Emerging Issues in Inflammatory Bowel Disease.* Falk Symposium 151. 2006
ISBN 978-1-4020-5701-4

152. Fockens P, Schulz H-J, Rösch T, Špičák J, eds. *Endoscopy 2006 – Update and Live Demonstration.* Falk Symposium 152. 2008   ISBN 978-1-4020-9147-6

153. Dignass A, Rachmilewitz D, Stange E-F, Weinstock JV, eds. *Immunoregulation in Inflammatory Bowel Diseases – Current Understanding and Innovation.* Falk Symposium 153. 2007   ISBN 978-1-4020-5888-2

154. Adler G, Fiocchi C, Lazebnik LB, Vorobiev GI, eds. *Inflammatory Bowel Disease – Diagnostic and Therapeutic Strategies.* Falk Symposium 154. 2007
ISBN 978-1-4020-6115-8

155. Keppler D, Beuers U, Leuschner U, Stiehl A, Trauner M, Paumgartner G, eds. *Bile Acids: Biological Actions and Clinical Relevance.* Falk Symposium 155. 2007
ISBN 978-1-4020-6251-3

156. Blum HE, Cox DW, Häussinger D, Jansen PLM, Kullak-Ublick GA, eds. *Genetics in Liver Diseases.* Falk Symposium 156. 2007   ISBN 978-14020-6393-0

157. Diehl AM, Hayashi N, Manns MP, Sauerbruch T, eds. *Chronic Hepatitis: Metabolic, Cholestatic, Viral and Autoimmune.* Falk Symposium 157. 2007
ISBN 978-1-4020-6522-4

158. Gasche G, Herrerías Gutiérrez JM, Gassull M, Monterio E, eds. *Intestinal Inflammation and Colorectal Cancer.* Falk Symposium 158. 2007
ISBN 978-1-4020-6825-6

159. Tözün N, Mantzaris G, Dağlı Ü, Schölmerich J, eds. *IBD 2007 – Achievements in Research and Clinical Practice.* Falk Symposium 159. 2008
ISBN 978-1-4020-6986-4

160. Ferkolj I, Gangl A, Galle PR, Vucelic B, eds. *Pathogenesis and Clinical Practice in Gastroenterology.* Falk Symposium 160. 2008   ISBN 978-1-4020-8766-0

161. Carey MC, Gabryelewicz A, Díte P, Keim V, Mössner J, eds. *Future Perspectives in Gastroenterology.* Falk Symposium 161. 2008   ISBN 978-1-4020-8832-2

162. Bosch J, Lammert F, Burroughs AK, Lebrec D, Sauerbruch T, eds. *Liver Cirrhosis: From Pathophysiology to Disease Management.* Falk Symposium 162. 2008
ISBN 978-1-4020-8655-7

163. Adler G, Fan D-M, Jia J-D, LaRusso NF, Owyang, C, eds. *Chronic Inflammation of Liver and Gut.* Falk Symposium 163. 2008   ISBN 978-1-4020-9352-4

164. Tulassay Z, Ditě P, Krejs GJ, Schölmerich J, Schultz H-J, eds. *Intestinal Disorders.* Falk Symposium 164. 2009   ISBN 978-1-4020-9590-0

165. Keppler D, Beuers U, Stiehl A, Trauner M, eds. *Bile Acid Biology and Therapeutic Actions.* Falk Symposium 165. 2009   ISBN 978-1-4020-9643-3

165A. Lieberman DA, Malfertheiner P, Riemann JF, Spechler SJ, eds. *Strategies of Cancer Prevention in Gastroenterology.* Falk Workshop. 2009
ISBN 978-90-481-2628-6

166. Ell C, Ponchon T, Riemann JF, Sakai P, Yamamoto H, eds. *GI Endoscopy – Standards and Innovations.* Falk Symposium 166. 2009   ISBN 978-90-481-2748-1

167. Day CP, Galle PR, Lohse AW, Thorgeirsson SS, eds. *Liver under Constant Attack – From Fat to Viruses.* Falk Symposium 167. 2009   ISBN 978-90-481-2758-0